Care of the Critically Ill Surgical Patient (CCrISP™)

Care of the Critically Ill Surgical Patient (CCrISP™)

2nd Edition

Edited by
Iain D. Anderson

Consultant Surgeon, Hope Hospital, Manchester, UK
Tutor in Surgical Critical Care,
The Royal College of Surgeons of England

A member of the
Hodder Headline Group
LONDON

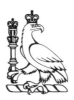

The Royal
College
of
Surgeons
of
England

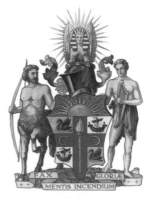

The Royal Australasian
College of Surgeons

First published in Great Britain in 2003 by
Arnold, a member of the Hodder Headline Group,
338 Euston Road, London NW1 3BH

http://www.arnoldpublishers.com

Distributed in the United States of America by
Oxford University Press Inc.,
198 Madison Avenue, New York, NY10016
Oxford is a registered trademark of Oxford University Press

British Library Cataloguing in Publication Data
A catalogue record for this book is available from the British Library

Library of Congress Cataloging-in-Publication Data
A catalog record for this book is available from the Library of Congress

ISBN   0 340 81048 3

2 3 4 5 6 7 8 9 10

Commissioning Editor: Serena Bureau
Development Editor: Layla Vandenbergh
Project Editor: Wendy Rooke
Production Controller: Deborah Smith
Cover Design: Stewart Larking

Typeset in 9 on 10 New Century Schoolbook by Phoenix Photosetting, Chatham, Kent
Printed and bound in Spain

What do you think about this book? Or any other Arnold title? Please send your comments to
feedback.arnold@hodder.co.uk

Contents

Contributors to the 2nd edition

Mr I D Anderson BSc MD FRCS
Consultant Surgeon, Hope Hospital,
Manchester, UK
(*Editor and Tutor in Surgical Critical Care,
The Royal College of Surgeons of England*)

Dr J R Goodall FRCA
Consultant in Anaesthetics and Intensive Care
Medicine, Hope Hospital, Manchester, UK

Dr M Hunter MB ChB FRACS
Consultant Surgeon and Intensivist and Senior
Lecturer in Surgery, Dunedin Hospital, Dunedin
School of Medicine, University of Otago,
New Zealand
(*Representative of the Royal Australasian College of
Surgeons*)

Dr B Riley MBE BSc FRCA
Consultant, Adult Intensive Care Unit,
Queen's Medical Centre, Nottingham, UK

Professor B J Rowlands MD FRCS FACS FRCSI
Professor of Surgery, University of Nottingham,
and Consultant Surgeon, Queen's Medical Centre,
Nottingham, UK
(*Chairman of Working Group*)

Mr R D Sayers MD FRCS
Consultant Vascular Surgeon, Royal Infirmary,
Leicester and Honorary Senior Lecturer in Surgery,
University of Leicester, Leicester, UK

Dr G B Smith FRCA FRCP
Consultant in Intensive Care Medicine,
Queen Alexandra Hospital, Portsmouth, UK

Professor M M Thompson MD FRCS
Professor of Surgery,
St George's Hospital Medical School,
London, UK

Mr G L Carlson MD FRCS
Consultant Surgeon, Hope Hospital,
Manchester, UK

Miss Shauntelle Hodel BsocSci
Project Co-ordinator, The Royal College of Surgeons
of England, UK

Acknowledgement

Mr A T King FRCS
Consultant Neurosurgeon, Hope Hospital,
Manchester, UK

Other Contributors to the 1st Edition

Dr T N Appleyard

Mrs O Egerton

Professor K C H Fearon

Mr D R Griffin

Professor D J Leaper

Dr G Ramsay

Mr R C G Russell

Professor J M Ryan

Dr A I K Short

Dr S W Turner

Dr R G Wheatley

Foreword to 1st Edition

On Saturday 15 April 1989, at a football match in the English city of Sheffield, an incident occurred in a tightly packed crowd which resulted in 96 mainly young people being crushed to death with many others seriously injured. The name of the football ground, Hillsborough, has become embedded in the English language as being synonymous with a major civilian disaster associated with needless loss of life. It would be difficult to see how anything positive could emerge from such a tragedy but there is a precedent, admittedly on a much smaller scale.

In 1976, in rural Nebraska, USA, a plane being piloted by an orthopaedic surgeon crashed. One of the six occupants was killed instantly and four were critically injured. The primary care received by the injured was judged by the doctors at the admitting hospital, and the orthopaedic surgeon himself, to be less than ideal. As a result the local surgeons decided that they should take some action to establish innovative training courses to help those unused to managing the seriously injured to deal with such cases. Thus arose the now well-recognised and respected Advanced Trauma Life Support (ATLS®) courses which use simulation and scene setting to mimic major injury and to improve the quality and realism or training.

In 1988 ATLS was introduced into the United Kingdom by The Royal College of Surgeons of England and became instantly popular with all those tasked with the management of the seriously injured, and there is no doubt that ATLS techniques were used at Hillsborough and may well have prevented an even higher death rate. Although difficult to prove scientifically there is virtually universal agreement that ATLS courses have improved care and contributed to the lowering of the death rate after road traffic accidents which has become such a marked feature of United Kingdom accident statistics of recent years. ATLS however deals only with the early stage of injury and there is undoubtedly a need for improvement in the management of that critical period following injury, during critical surgical illness, or after major surgery where patients may be in intensive therapy or high dependency units.

The educational techniques used in ATLS® are equally applicable in critical care training. Iain Anderson and his colleagues, with the help of the Education Department at The Royal College of Surgeons of England and the support of the Hillsborough Charity, have produced a course, similar in concept to ATLS and using its techniques, dealing with the management of the critically ill surgical patient. This book is produced in a format that will enable the text to be used either independently or alongside the course. This innovative approach has the potential for improving the care of critically ill patients in the same manner and to the same degree as that achieved by ATLS.

The book deals concisely and clearly with the whole range of issues associated with the critically ill, including the management of the psychological problems which were such an issue after Hillsborough. The surgical trainees who undergo this course and read this textbook will have restored to them the confidence once felt by all surgical trainees in the management of the critically ill. This confidence was based on the famous textbook by the American surgeon Francis Moore, *The Metabolic Care of the Surgical Patient*, a book that is widely accepted as being the foundation stone of modern intensive care.

I hope those so tragically bereaved at Hillsborough will regard this book and its accompanying course as a living addition to the more permanent memorial in Liverpool to those who died.

Sir Miles Irving DSc (Hon.) MD ChM FRCS
FACS (Hon.) FMedSci
Emeritus Professor of Surgery
University of Manchester
Chairman of Newcastle upon Tyne
Hospitals NHS Trust

Preface

Critical care is now an accepted part of surgical practice. Within the last few years it has become part of postgraduate exams; more importantly, it is part of the everyday practice of the majority of practising surgeons. This includes responsibility for critically ill surgical patients, whether they are on the ward, in surgical high dependency units or intensive care units. Consequently, surgeons in training must quickly develop their own skills to enable them to look after these patients following an emergency admission, major surgery or unexpected complication. They must also be able to function effectively with colleagues from related disciplines, particularly anaesthesia and intensive care.

This book, like its predecessor, is the manual of the Care of the Critically Ill Surgical Patient (CCrISP) Course of The Royal College of Surgeons of England. The CCrISP course was established in 1996 by a multidisciplinary working group with a grant from the Hillsborough Disaster Fund. This fund was raised from public subscription following the Hillsborough football stadium disaster in 1989. Since 1996, the CCrISP course has found a key role in training junior surgeons on account of its success and popularity. It is highly recommended that all basic surgical trainees in England and Wales sit the course, and it is compulsory for such trainees in Australasia. The course is available in over 50 centres, including Ireland, Scotland and Hong Kong.

The CCrISP course aims to assist doctors in training to learn the skills necessary to look after critically ill surgical patients. The theoretical basis of the course is laid out in this book, together with illustrative case scenarios, guidelines for management and the system of approach successfully advocated by the course. The course itself reinforces the clinical application of the theory base and also places emphasis on the acquisition of practical skills, improved patient management and the development of the interpersonal skills needed to relate to patients and colleagues alike. This practical guide is not an exhaustive text, but the practical guidance offered has proved of value to many surgical trainees at basic and higher levels. The need to master these skills becomes pressing as surgeons prepare to enter the registrar grade. This is the stage where they will take on more responsibility for assessment, decision-making and ultimately operating on patients with serious conditions. The process of acquiring these skills is stressful for trainees and potentially so for patients and trainers as well. The CCrISP course also aims to help the trainee develop mechanisms to make this change as smoothly as possible.

This current review is based on the experience and recommendations of the many instructors and candidates who have sat the course over the last few years. The approaches advocated are based on accepted modern consensus practice, and the revision has again been conducted by a multidisciplinary group with input from the UK and Australasia.

I hope you find it of value.

Iain D Anderson BSc MD FRCS
Consultant Surgeon, Hope Hospital,
Manchester, UK
Tutor in Surgical Critical Care,
The Royal College of Surgeons of England

Acknowledgements

The establishment of the Care of the Critically Ill Surgical Patient (CCrISP) course and manual was assisted by a generous donation from the Hillsborough Disaster Fund, and the CCrISP programme is now supported by Jane and Leon Grant.

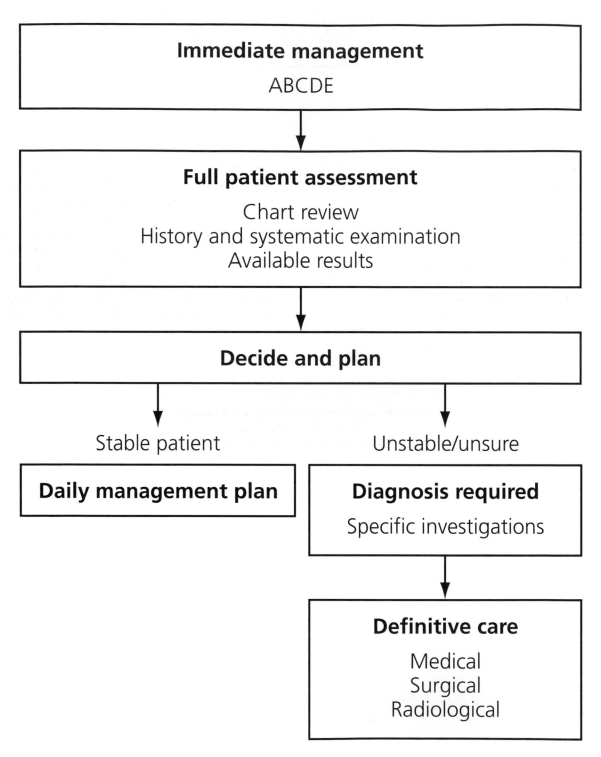

CCrISP system of patient assessment

CCrISP course objectives

- Develop the theoretical basis and practical skills necessary to manage the critically ill surgical patient
- Be able to assess critically ill patients accurately and appreciate the value of a system of assessment for the critically ill
- Understand the subtlety and variety of presentation of critical illness and the methods available for improving detection
- Understand the importance of a plan of action in order to achieve clinical progress, accurate diagnosis and early definitive treatment. Be able to formulate a plan of action and involve appropriate assistance in a timely manner

- Appreciate that complications tend to occur in a cascade and realise that prevention of complications is fundamental to successful outcome
- Be aware of the support facilities available and interact with nursing staff, other surgeons and intensivists/anaesthetists, being aware, in particular, of the surgeon's role in the delivery of multidisciplinary care to the critically ill
- Understand the requirements of the patient and their relatives during critical illness and be able to inform and support both appropriately

> **Success depends upon attention to detail**
> *Joseph Lister 1827–1912*
> **A stitch in time saves nine**
> *Traditional*

Abbreviations

ABG	arterial blood gas	ECG	electrocardiogram
ACE	angiotensin-converting enzyme	ECLS	extracorporeal life support
ADH	antidiuretic hormone	EEG	electroencephalogram
A&E	accident and emergency	EIA	epidural infusion analgesia
AF	atrial fibrillation	ENT	ear, nose and throat
AP	anteroposterior	ERCP	endoscopic retrograde
ARDS	acute respiratory distress syndrome		cholangiopancreatography
ASB	assisted spontaneous breathing		
ATLS	Advanced Trauma Life Support	FAST	focused abdominal sonography in
AV	atrioventricular		trauma
		FBC	full blood count
BAL	bronchial alveolar lavage	FEV_1	forced expiratory volume in 1 s
BBB	bundle branch block	FRC	functional residual capacity
BCAA	branched-chain amino acid	FTc	corrected flow time
BE	base excess		
BLS	basic life support	GABA	gamma-aminobutyric acid
BMI	body mass index	GCS	Glasgow coma scale
BSA	body surface area	GI	gastrointestinal
CCF	congestive cardiac failure	HDU	high dependency unit
CCrISP	Care of the Critically Ill Surgical	HIV	human immunodeficiency virus
	Patient	5-HT	5-hydroxytryptamine (serotonin)
CI	cardiac index		
CNS	central nervous system	IAP	intra-abdominal pressure
COAD	chronic obstructive airways disease	ICU	intensive care unit
COX-2	cyclo-oxygenase 2	ICP	intracranial pressure
CPAP	continuous positive airway pressure	IgE	immunoglobulin E
CPP	cerebral perfusion pressure	IHD	ischaemic heart disease
CPR	cardiopulmonary resuscitation	IVNAA	in vivo neutron activation analysis
CRF	chronic renal failure	IVU	intravenous urogram
CSM	carotid sinus massage		
CT	computed tomography	JVP	jugular venous pressure
CTZ	chemoreceptor trigger zone		
CVP	central venous pressure	LAP	left atrial pressure
CVS	cardiovascular system	LFT	liver function test
CXR	chest X-ray	LVEDP	left ventricular end diastolic pressure
		LVEDV	left ventricular end diastolic volume
DPL	diagnostic peritoneal lavage	LVF	left ventricular failure
DVT	deep vein thrombosis		
		MAP	mean arterial pressure
ECF	extracellular fluid	MI	myocardial infarction

MOF	multiple organ failure	PSV	pressure-support ventilation
MRI	magnetic resonance imaging	PTC	percutaneous transhepatic cholangiography
MRSA	methicillin-resistant *Staphylococcus aureus*	PTSD	post-traumatic stress disorder
NCA	nurse-controlled analgesia	RRT	renal replacement therapy
NICE	National Institute for Clinical Excellence	SHO	senior house officer
NSAID	non-steroidal anti-inflammatory drug	SIMV	synchronised intermittent mandatory ventilation
OSA	obstructive sleep apnoea	SIRS	systemic inflammatory response syndrome
PA	posteroanterior	SVC	superior vena cava
PAOP	pulmonary artery occlusion pressure	SVR	systemic vascular resistance
PAP	pulmonary artery pressure	SVT	supraventricular tachycardia
PCA	patient-controlled analgesia		
PCIRV	pressure-controlled inverse ratio ventilation	TNF	tumour necrosis factor
		TOD	transoesophageal Doppler
PCV	pressure-controlled ventilation		
PCWP	pulmonary capillary wedge pressure	VF	ventriculation fibrillation
PE	pulmonary embolism	VT	ventricular tachycardia
PEEP	positive end expiratory pressure		
PEM	protein–energy malnutrition	WPW	Wolff–Parkinson–White syndrome
PiCCO	pulse contour cardiac output with indicator dilution		

Introduction **1**

Looking after critically ill surgical patients successfully is a major and, at times, stressful part of a surgeon's life. Surgical practice is dynamic and as changes to hospital practice occur, they may help or hinder other aspects of the delivery of care. Some of the current factors are shown in Table 1.1.

Table 1.1 *Risk and stress factors in surgical critical care*

Ageing population

Concomitant disease processes

Complexity of surgery

Higher standards of monitoring

Greater number of postoperative interventions and therapies

Expectations by patients, relatives and staff

Shortage of permanent and experienced nurses

Shortened duty hours for junior surgeons and different on-call
 arrangements

Many surgical patients are old and/or sick, have undergone major surgery or have been admitted as an emergency. With modern duty arrangements, you will often be responsible for this type of patient from other surgical teams, and you may well be on duty with junior and senior staff with whom you work only occasionally. Consequently, the duty surgeon will be faced frequently with critically ill surgical patients with whom they are not familiar. The establishment of high dependency units (HDUs) has been an undoubted advance, but not all unwell patients can be cared for in HDUs; in any case, patient care in HDUs often remains the responsibility of the surgical team. Furthermore, the HDU can be a daunting place to those unfamiliar with it. The Care of the Critically Ill Surgical Patient (CCrISP) programme of The Royal College of Surgeons of England provides practical training to support the junior doctor who is faced with managing unwell surgical patients today. In particular, the course provides a simple, safe and accepted approach with which you can begin to assess and manage every patient you encounter, no matter how complex.

The capacity of surgical patients to withstand surgery and any complications depends on their age, underlying disease process and any coexisting illnesses. Once a surgical patient develops multiple organ failure (and therefore requires intensive care unit (ICU) support), overall mortality can be around 50%. It is clear, therefore, that detecting and treating problems **before** this stage is reached is the most preferable course of action. Unfortunately, critical surgical illness can often be detected easily only once a relatively advanced stage has been reached. The challenge for all surgeons who deal with patients who may become critically ill is to develop a system of practice that will allow the **identification and correction of complications at the earliest stage**. Improvements can be achieved through three mechanisms:

- prediction: identifying an at-risk population;
- prevention; and
- prompt identification and early adequate treatment.

These mechanisms are complementary and will apply in differing proportions to different patient groups. These strategies in surgical critical care are at least as important as the heroic but often unsuccessful rescue of the patient who has reached a state of extremis.

AIM OF TRAINING IN SURGICAL CRITICAL CARE

Restricting the perception of a critically ill surgical patient to the patient with multiple organ failure dying in the ICU is an almost pointless exercise. Critical illness begins, is **detectable and is treatable** long before this, and the aim of this manual and the CCrISP course is to equip you to predict, prevent and treat these illnesses accordingly. Likewise, it will be difficult to offer best care to emergency cases or to unfit patients upon whom you conduct major surgery without the necessary management skills for ward and HDU practice. Traditionally, surgical training has focused on pathology and operative surgical treatment, but with the advances in critical care techniques and changes in patient demographics, more structured teaching in the nonoperative management of critically ill patients is essential.

AIM OF THE CCrISP COURSE

To improve practical management of critically ill surgical patients:

- clinical method
- practical skills
- communication and organisational skills
- focused knowledge.

Too many deaths and unplanned admissions to ICU occur because appropriate, thoughtful and early action was not taken. Studies show that some 30–40% of patients admitted to ICU received suboptimal care on the ward at some stage. Together with the CCrISP course, this book aims to make you think about the ill or potentially ill patient. It will help you to identify the patient who may become ill and take the necessary steps: to prevent that patient developing complications; to deal with any emergency arising on the ward; to assess and respond to the immediate problem; and to initiate treatment while awaiting specialist help. Following immediate management, you will learn the importance of identifying and correcting the underlying cause. Many adverse episodes can be terminated by the immediate provision of **simple support** (*eg* oxygen, fluids) and by the early attainment of a diagnosis so **early definitive treatment** can be instituted (*eg* antibiotics, provision of usual cardiac medications, drainage of an abscess).

Practice point

Prompt, simple actions save lives and prevent complications.

Avoidable problems occur because these simple manoeuvres are not taken or, more commonly, because the effectiveness and adequacy of such manoeuvres are not checked and further effective steps not taken. For example, failure to institute and ensure effective support for an elderly patient with retained pulmonary secretions on a Saturday may result in established pneumonia by Monday morning. Survival may be threatened and length of stay will certainly be prolonged (see Case history 1.1).

Case history 1.1

A 68-year-old man, a smoker with mild chronic airways disease, underwent laparotomy for a perforated duodenal ulcer on Monday night. An epidural was placed but was removed on day four (Friday). He received chest physiotherapy during the week, but no specific request was made for weekend treatment. His team was not on call and, because he seemed to be progressing, no formal handover was made. On Saturday afternoon, he was noted to be in pain and to have a tachypnoea. The house officer was called, but he was busy and did not see the patient until 9pm, by which time the patient was pyrexial. A course of ciprofloxacin was prescribed (although none would be available from pharmacy until 9am), and the senior house officer (SHO) was informed. The patient was reviewed at the end of the on-call ward round late on Sunday morning. He was found to be considerably worsened, with pyrexia, dyspnoea and bronchial breathing. He was started on monitored oxygen and nebulisers, and urgent chest physiotherapy was arranged, following review of his requirements for analgesia. He took 10 days to get over the pneumonia and his hospital stay was prolonged by about two weeks.

Learning points

- The best critical care is simple and preventive; late, heroic interventions are less successful.
- Prompt, simple actions save lives and prevent complications.
- Make, use and update action plans.
- Success depends upon attention to detail.

Implementing simple interventions such as the above requires the same combination of skills as do more complex or dramatic episodes in surgical critical care. These skills include clinical examination, judicious investigation, formulation of a plan of action, institution thereof (including the necessary communication with colleagues and practical techniques) and re-evaluation of the patient with, if necessary, the ability to invoke greater degrees of support at the right time. These skills, together with relevant practical procedures and the related base knowledge, will be taught and assessed in simulated clinical situations during the CCrISP course, the emphasis throughout being on practical management of common problems. However, there is no reason why you cannot adopt a systematic approach to your own practice directly.

> **Practice point**
> Reassess! Has your intervention been effective? Further, prompt, simple actions may be necessary.

WHAT THIS MANUAL IS NOT

Neither this manual nor the CCrISP course will teach you to become a specialist in intensive care. Instead, the main thrust is about prevention of further deterioration through accurate and prompt assessment and treatment to avoid complications on the ward and in the HDU. However, there does exist a considerable overlap between the practical skills and approaches to care seen in the ICU and in the surgical HDU, and junior surgeons benefit greatly from a period spent working in the ICU. Surgeons must be aware of the nature and principles of intensive care, the support available there and the time when such support should be sought. They must also be aware of the limitations of the ICU and the nature of support that the surgical team must provide to the ICU team when their patients are being treated in an ICU. During your training, you will need to develop an appreciation of the surgical needs of patients in the ICU, the difficulties of assessment there, and the impact of ICU care on your patients and their disease processes. Following discharge from the ICU, a further range of skills is necessary to ensure that the patient does not fall into the trap of early deterioration and readmission to an ICU. These topics will be dealt with and will contribute towards making you a better practitioner of surgical critical care.

This manual takes a practical, management-oriented approach to critical care. It is not designed to be a comprehensive text of surgical critical care and you may wish to supplement your reading with such.

CONTINUUM OF CARE

There is a continuum of care from the ICU through the HDU and the ward to the community, each providing different attributes of importance to success-

ful surgical care. Compared with surgical wards, the HDU is an area of enhanced nurse/patient ratios (1:2), with appropriate monitoring equipment (arterial pressure, central venous pressure (CVP), pulse oximetry, heart rate) and accumulated nursing expertise in both critical illness and specialist surgical care. Patients are usually within 24–72 hours of operation and either are at high risk of complications or have developed a complication or impairment of vital organ function on account of their illness, surgery or coexisting medical disease. Some HDUs will manage patients with single organ failure, but the main aim is to detect and prevent further deterioration.

By way of contrast, the ICU offers more intensive nursing ratios, monitoring and support, and care is usually directed by ICU medical staff in collaboration with the patient's surgical team. Here, failed organ systems can be supported by complex interventions (eg ventilation, high-dose or multiple inotrope therapy, haemofiltration, dialysis). ICU staff may be less experienced than their HDU counterparts in the surgical aspects of management of patients following complex procedures.

Although the precise profile of patients in different critical care units will vary between hospitals, you should note that many patients will require surgical and ICU-type input whichever type of bed they are in. Surgeons have a role to play in the care of patients on the ICU, and ICU staff often help to manage patients on the ward. The proportion of care needed from each team will vary with time and with the patient's immediate needs (see Fig. 1.1). The HDU

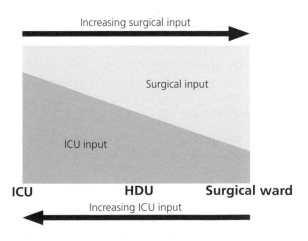

Figure 1.1 *Changing requirements for critical support in surgical patients*

occupies a middle ground in terms of the balance between management of surgical problems and the management of systemic or multiorgan problems.

Special surgical units (*eg* transplant units) offer varying combinations of facilities. Assessing and managing patients there will require specialist knowledge and techniques, but most of the immediate management relies on the same basic principles. Indeed, many complex problems in critical care can be broken down, assessed and treated in a similar manner.

PATIENTS TO BE CONSIDERED

In caring for critically ill surgical patients, three categories of patients can be discerned (see Table 1.2):

* the routine preoperative patient,
* the emergency admission, and
* the ward patient.

Table 1.2 *Patients at risk and risk practices*

Patients at risk

Emergencies

Elderly

Coexisting disease processes

Non-progressing patient

Severity of acute illness or magnitude of operation

Massive transfusion

Rebleeding

Failure/delay to diagnose and treat underlying problem

Already developed another complication

Established shock state

Risk practices

Incomplete or infrequent assessment

Failure to act on abnormal findings

Failure to ensure that interventions have been successful

Failure of continuity of care (poor communication)

Failure of nursing support (insufficient numbers or
   expertise) – wrong ward

The preoperative patient

Patients on steroids for severe chronic airways disease, for example, present obvious risks. Here, a balance must be struck between the necessity of operation and the individual risks. Careful specialist and anaesthetic assessment, if not obtained already, will be needed, and plans will have to be made for postoperative care. Less obvious problems may act synergistically, but a similar approach can minimise their effects (see Case history 1.2).

Case history 1.2

Take, for example, the patient for inguinal hernia repair who appears fit but who has left bundle branch block, a smoker's cough, mild alcoholic liver disease and prostatism. After operation, a predictable chain of minor events may ultimately prove fatal: simple hernia repair leads to urinary retention; subsequent urine infection contributes to a confusional state; failure of expectoration causes atelectasis and then a chest infection; underlying ischaemic heart disease cannot cope with hypoxia. The patient arrests 'suddenly' on day three on the short-stay ward.

The patient was great company at the golf club, and your position on the club's waiting list will not be helped by the perceptions of his erstwhile partners:

'Poor old Joe – doctor said he died suddenly.'

'He wasn't himself at visiting time – you'd have thought they would have picked something up in time.'

'Not so good, eh? Just had a hernia – sort of thing they do as a day case.'

The emergency admission

Emergency admissions present with a wide range of underlying diseases and an equal spectrum of comorbid conditions, ranging from the unrecognised (*eg* occult ischaemic heart disease) to the obvious (*eg* anticoagulation), which complicate matters. Many patients undergoing emergency major surgery are inherently unstable and easy prey to further complications. Preventing these complications begins by achieving prompt and effective resuscitation and surgery – no easy matter in an elderly group presenting out of normal working hours. Anaesthesia removes vascular tone and can cause catastrophic hypotension in the hypovolaemic patient. It is obvious that you cannot do a laparotomy on a patient with peritonitis until they are resuscitated, but a patient with a fractured neck of femur also requires careful resuscitation. On the other hand, you must identify the bleeding patient who needs simultaneous surgery and resuscitation. Co-ordinating appropriate care following surgery, especially out of routine hours, can tax your organisational and communication skills. Clear guidelines must be given to nursing staff, and regular medical review must be undertaken.

The routine ward round

On business ward rounds, you will review all your patients. This is probably the most important way in which you practise good critical care. By conducting a logical and thorough round, you can prevent or identify many problems and get them corrected before they cause significant upset. The system of assessment and formulation of management plans described in Chapter 2 applies to these patients every bit as much as to those who are obviously unwell.

The ward patient with complications

Patients who develop obvious complications present similar challenges to those of the emergency admissions, the major pitfall being a failure to take further prompt action when initial interventions are not sufficiently successful.

More difficult are patients who 'fail to progress'. Here, there is usually an underlying problem eluding detection. These patients are often elderly, and the recognition of the subtle sign can lead to appropriate action preventing major problems arising, as indicated in Case history 1.2.

METHOD OF APPROACH

Basic surgical trainees, like house officers or junior residents, are essentially data-gatherers: they pass information to seniors. As you progress in seniority, your role changes. When you progress to being a registrar, you become much more of a decision-maker, making critical decisions constantly, on ward rounds or about emergencies, which will have a direct bearing on patient outcome. Of course, you will have senior colleagues to discuss things with, but nevertheless there is a marked change in role and responsibility at this stage. Using the skills and approaches described in this manual and on the CCrISP course will help you to appreciate some of the changes that you need to undergo. These will help the change to be less stressful and more successful for all.

All clinicians find the management of emergencies stressful at times, and this is usually contributed to by lack of information (about the patient, their diseases or recent events), disorganisation and initial lack of appreciation of the severity of the situation. You will, by now, have experienced episodes in your own practice of critical illness that were not managed as well as they might have been. It is useful at this stage to reflect on the reasons why those suboptimal events occurred.

The aim now is to build on your present knowledge and experience, to train you to think, to be in command of any situation by rapidly assessing the situation and the patient, responding to the immediate problem and initiating treatment. Certain simple immediate thoughts can help set your assessment off on the right foot.

THINKING ON THE RUN
- Think early – when the telephone call comes:
  - instructions to caller
  - what do I know about ...?
    what will I do when I arrive?
- Think basics – when I arrive:
  - check and secure the ABCs
  - what system fails?
  - what observations are available?
    what observations can I make quickly?
- Think simply:
  - how quickly must I act?
  - do I have a diagnosis?
  - how will I get that diagnosis safely?
  - What help do I need?

The CCrISP programme will emphasise some quite basic clinical and scientific concepts: those that clinicians experienced in this field employ in frontline practice. Above all, it will help you to think straight when you are under pressure in the clinical arena. It will provide you with mechanisms that will facilitate successful care, the most important of which is a systematic means by which to assess a critically ill surgical patient. Until now, you will have approached problems by taking a detailed history and then examining the patient. However, critically ill patients require a system that lets you identify and treat problems rapidly, according to priority and as you assess the patient further. This approach is detailed in Chapter 2.

SUMMARY

- **Preventing** deterioration is more effective than attempting salvage at a later stage.
- The scope of surgical critical care includes the prediction and prevention of problems as well as the investigation of and intervention in the acutely unwell patient.
- Surgical critical care extends downwards from the HDU to the ward level (prediction, prevention) and upwards to integrate with the ICU, *ie* a **continuum of care** exists.
- **Simple**, logical thoughts and **actions** will often be effective.

Assessing the critically ill 2 surgical patient

Objectives

This chapter will help you to:

- Assess and manage critically ill patients systematically.
- Recognise the critically ill patient who must undergo simultaneous examination and resuscitation when first seen.
- Recognise that examination and resuscitation must be performed in a systematic manner,

treating life-threatening problems in the order of their threat to life.
- Be aware of the importance of identifying and correcting the underlying abnormality.
- Formulate daily management plans for patients on critical care units.

INTRODUCTION

Surgical patients requiring critical care fall into two broad groups. First, there are those who are acutely unwell, having been newly admitted or having suffered an acute deterioration on the ward. These patients require **simultaneous resuscitation**, **diagnosis** and then **definitive treatment**.

Second, there are those patients already on the ward or within an HDU who require re-evaluation and formulation of a management plan on at least a twice-daily basis. Here, the aim is to ensure that the patient is progressing, *ie* getting better. It is better to prevent morbidity by detecting problems as early as possible; failure to progress is an important sign that an incipient problem is present. If you fail to diagnose and treat that problem until it has produced a major deterioration in the patient's condition, then the patient's likelihood of survival is reduced dramatically.

The approach to the assessment of the sick surgical patient should be **systematic** to ensure that life-threatening or potentially life-threatening conditions and important aspects of care are not overlooked. Employing a system regularly ensures that you will use it when you are under pressure. The suggested system of assessment is shown in Fig. 2.1. This is the system that many experienced doctors use. The

same system is used for all patients, regardless of whether they are stable or unstable.

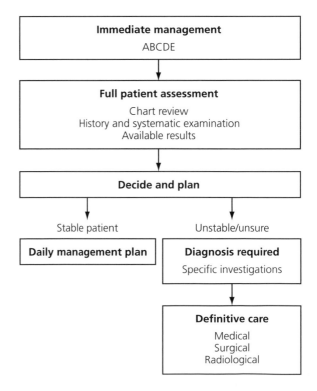

Figure 2.1 *The CCrISP system of assessment*

IMMEDIATE ASSESSMENT AND TREATMENT OF THE ACUTELY ILL PATIENT

When assessing the acutely ill patient, your goal is to determine what is making the patient ill and, having identified any life-threatening problem, to treat it immediately. Life-threatening illnesses kill in a predictable and reproducible pattern. When viewed in isolation, a disease process that produces an obstructed airway will kill more quickly than one that produces direct lung dysfunction, which in turn kills more quickly than isolated haemorrhage or cardiac dysfunction. Many critically ill surgical patients have linked abnormalities of more than one vital system. Hence, it is important not to be distracted by obvious but minor factors and to assess and treat problems systematically.

Immediate management

A – airway assessment and treatment
B – breathing assessment and treatment
C – circulation assessment and treatment
D – dysfunction of the central nervous system
E – exposure of the patient sufficient for full assessment and treatment

This process prioritises the order in which assessment and treatment is carried out. Although it is represented as a sequence, such information can often be obtained virtually simultaneously. For example, the patient's response to the question 'How are you?' can be very revealing: if the patient is able to reply in a coherent manner, this suggests that, at least for the moment, the patient is in control of their airway sufficiently to allow an adequate intake of breath, adequate respiratory function to produce oxygen transfer, adequate circulatory function to perfuse the brain, and adequate central nervous system function to formulate a reply. While this is encouraging, it does not release you from the need to perform a detailed assessment of each of the ABCDE components of the immediate assessment.

Practice point

Be alert to the risks of hepatitis and human immunodeficiency virus (HIV).

Always be alert to the risks of blood-borne diseases. In almost all emergencies, there is time and facility to adopt safety measures.

A – AIRWAY

Recognition that airway obstruction is present is based on a simple 'look, listen and feel' clinical assessment:

- Look for the presence of central cyanosis, obstructed 'seesaw' pattern of respiration or abdominal breathing, use of accessory muscles of respiration, tracheal tug, alteration of level of consciousness and any obvious obstruction by foreign body or vomitus.
- Listen for abnormal sounds, such as grunting, snoring, gurgling, hoarseness or stridor.
- Feel for airflow on inspiration and expiration.

If objective signs of airway obstruction are present, then the immediate goals are to obtain and secure the airway to provide for adequate oxygenation. **Immediate** intervention is required to prevent hypoxic brain damage, so administer high-flow oxygen (12–15 l/min, preferably via a reservoir bag).

Often, only simple methods are required to obtain an airway, such as chin lift or jaw thrust to open the airway, suction to remove secretions, the insertion of an oral Guedel airway, if tolerated, or a soft nasopharyngeal airway if the gag reflex is present.

If such methods are not successful, then a definitive airway (a cuffed tube secured in the trachea) is required. Such endotracheal tubes may be passed orally or nasally, but the oral route with the larynx visualised by direct laryngoscopy using a laryngoscope is the most usual choice. If the patient is in extremis, then this may be accomplished without the use of drugs, but where the patient is responsive and endotracheal intubation is indicated, you *must* seek help from an anaesthetist. Attempts at intubation without first pre-oxygenating the patient are futile and dangerous. If endotracheal intubation is unsuccessful, then a surgical airway should be performed, with cricothyroidotomy being the treatment of choice.

Remember that patients can be maintained with an airway plus bag-and-mask ventilation as required while waiting for the anaesthetist. This is often a better option for the non-expert, particularly within a hospital, where skilled help is usually available rapidly.

Protect the airway. Patients who are not fully conscious may have an airway that they cannot protect and that is patent only intermittently. These patients may tolerate and benefit from airway manoeuvres while the cause of their reduced conscious level is addressed.

If there is a risk of coexisting pathology of the cervical spine, than all airway manoeuvres should be performed while maintaining manual in-line immobilisation of the cervical spine.

B – BREATHING

Objective evidence of respiratory distress or inadequate ventilation can also be determined using the clinical 'look, listen and feel' technique:

- Look for central cyanosis, use of accessory muscles of respiration, respiratory rate, equality and depth of respiration, sweating, raised jugular venous pressure (JVP), patency of any chest drains and the presence of any paradoxical abdominal movement. Note the inspired oxygen concentration (FiO$_2$) and saturation if pulse oximetry is in use, but remember that pulse oximetry does **not** detect hypercapnia.
- Listen for noisy breathing, clearance of secretions by coughing, ability of the patient to talk in complete sentences (evidence of confusion or decreased level of consciousness may indicate hypoxia or hypercapnia, respectively) and auscultate for abnormal breath sounds, heart sounds and rhythm.
- Feel for equality of chest movement, position of trachea, the presence of surgical emphysema or crepitus, paradoxical respiration and tactile vocal fremitus if indicated. Percuss the chest superiorly and laterally. Abdominal distension may limit diaphragmatic movement and in this respect is part of respiratory assessment.

The precise resuscitative treatment will be determined by the cause of the respiratory embarrassment and is discussed in Chapter 3. During the immediate assessment, you should look specifically for signs of the immediately life-threatening conditions of tension pneumothorax, massive haemothorax, open pneumothorax, flail chest and cardiac tamponade *and then treat these accordingly immediately*. Consider also the diagnoses of bronchial obstruction, bronchoconstriction, pulmonary embolism, cardiac failure (see C – circulation) and uncon-

sciousness (see D – dysfunction of the central nervous system) and, if present, treat them. Simple manoeuvres such as sitting the patient upright can help, but if the patient is tiring to the point of incipient respiratory arrest you will have to assist ventilation by bagging them, in conjunction with whatever airway manoeuvres have been necessary, until help arrives.

C – CIRCULATION

Hypovolaemia should always be considered to be the primary cause of circulatory dysfunction in the surgical patient until proved otherwise, and haemorrhage (overt or covert) must be excluded rapidly. Unless there are obvious signs of cardiogenic shock (in particular, raised JVP) you should regard *any* patient who is cool and tachycardic to have hypovolaemic shock, so establish and secure adequate venous access (at least one large (16G) cannula), send off blood for cross-matching and other routine tests, and initiate appropriate fluid replacement starting with a rapid fluid challenge of 10 ml/kg of warmed crystalloid in the normotensive patient or 20 ml/kg if the patient is hypotensive. Patients with known heart failure should receive an initial bolus of 5 ml/kg (unless you suspect that their current problem is pulmonary oedema) and closer monitoring may be needed.

Having identified and treated airway and breathing abnormalities that can compromise the circulation, life-threatening circulatory dysfunction is recognised by looking for:

- reduced peripheral perfusion (pallor, coolness, collapsed or underfilled veins – remember that blood pressure may be **normal** in the shocked patient);
- obvious external haemorrhage from wounds or drains;
- evidence of concealed haemorrhage:
  - thoracic or abdominal, even when an empty drain is present
  - into the gut or from pelvic or femoral fractures
  - alteration of level of consciousness secondary to cerebral underperfusion.

Initially, you should assess perfusion rather than blood pressure and institute management based on your findings as a priority. Check the blood pressure at an early point, but remember that it can often be preserved in a patient with significant circulatory problems. Marked hypotension is a late sign that needs rapid correction.

Feel for pulses, both peripheral and central, assessing for rate, quality, regularity and equality.

Treatment and monitoring are covered in detail in Chapters 5 and 6 but should be directed at haemorrhage control and restoration of tissue perfusion. You must remember that no amount of fluid replacement will be of use in the face of ongoing severe haemorrhage. **Immediate surgery** to control haemorrhage may be required at this stage as the only effective form of resuscitation; more frequently, urgent surgery will be needed to stop lesser degrees of continued haemorrhage.

Shocked patients fall into three categories:

- The obviously exsanguinating patient who needs **immediate** definitive treatment (usually surgery) to save their life.
- The unstable patient who needs rapid resuscitation and repeated reassessment over a short period while the cause is identified and treated. The patient may appear to respond transiently to aggressive fluid resuscitation. Urgent definitive treatment is essential.
- The patient with a relatively minor problem who responds rapidly and adequately to a fluid challenge and who remains stable on reassessment.

Reassessment (which occurs continuously in the initial stages) simply determines whether the patient is responding to the treatment. Clearly, if there is no response or only a transient or inadequate response, then different treatment is needed immediately. Patients requiring large and ongoing volumes of infusion are **not** stable, even if you can maintain reasonable vital signs.

The fluid challenge can be repeated and colloid solutions can be used provided you are aware of their different distribution and side effects (see Chapter 5). Only occasionally is it necessary to give uncross-matched blood, as type-specific blood is relatively safe and can be obtained within 10–20 minutes. Blood is presently the best resuscitation fluid for the bleeding patient who has cardiovascular instability and who requires, as a guide, more than 1500–2000 ml of resuscitation fluid.

Avoid blindly continuing to transfuse the patient who in reality **needs surgery**. Bleeding patients who need immediate surgery are encountered on the ward at least as frequently as in the emergency room; patients with postoperative bleeding or recurrent bleeding from a peptic ulcer who are pale and shocked are typical examples. As you resuscitate these patients, you should be calling for senior help, cross-matching eight units of blood, and alerting theatre, the anaesthetist and the porters. Shocked or hypotensive patients who are not bleeding are also seen regularly; again, do not continue to blindly fill up a patient with litres of fluid without a clear diagnosis, a clear plan or senior review (preferably all three).

Most surgeons have failed to respond adequately to continuing haemorrhage at some point during their career, so **reassess**, reconsider and do not leave a patient with inadequate perfusion without further adequate treatment.

Practice point

Most unwell surgical patients benefit from administration of oxygen and fluids while further assessment is undertaken. Reassess as resuscitation proceeds: it often takes more than one assessment to decide what the problem is.

D – DYSFUNCTION OF THE CENTRAL NERVOUS SYSTEM

In the initial assessment, a rapid assessment of neurological status is performed by examining the pupils and by following the AVPU system:

A – alert
V – responds to verbal stimulus
P – responds only to pain
U – unresponsive to any stimulus

You should remember that the surgical patient may have an alteration of conscious level due to causes other than a primary brain injury. **Hypoxia** with or without **hypercapnia** and cerebral underperfusion due to **shock** should have been detected already. Recent administration of sedatives, analgesics or anaesthetic drugs may be responsible. Hypoglycaemia is a common and sometimes overlooked cause that you should look for and treat. If you have thought of all these and the patient is still not fully conscious, review the ABCs: you might have missed something.

E – EXPOSURE

In order to make accurate diagnoses and allow access to the patient for therapeutic manoeuvres, it is essential that the patient is exposed adequately. You should be aware that not only does this allow the patient to become cold, but that it also exposes them to the view of others and that the patient's dignity must be respected.

End of immediate management

By the end of the phase of immediate assessment and management, you should have a patient who is showing signs of improvement and progressing out of immediate danger. You will very likely have called for help, and the patient may even have been to theatre or moved to the ICU before this point is reached.

By this stage, the patient should be receiving oxygen and intravenous fluids. Attach a pulse oximeter, check the blood pressure and check that the saturation (SaO_2) is above 94%. Arrange pressing investigations, such as gases, chest X-ray (CXR) or electrocardiography (ECG), insert a urinary catheter if appropriate and, if necessary, alert senior colleagues if you have not already done so. Before you start the next phase, quickly reassess the ABCs.

> **Practice point**
> If at any time during the immediate assessment the patient's condition deteriorates, you must reassess the ABCs.

Having initiated resuscitative manoeuvres, it will often take a few minutes for their effects to be apparent. Vital signs may not yet be normal, but provided the patient's condition is improving, you should use the time to continue with the next stage of assessment in order to determine the underlying cause of deterioration. Patients and their problems differ, so this system is an outline, not an immutable series of commands. However, if the patient is not improving, then reassess swiftly, get help and arrange for further immediate treatment.

Assessment of the 'stable' surgical patient

In many surgical patients, particularly during ward rounds, the vital signs will be normal. Often, this can be determined simply by looking at the patient, by asking how they are and by asking the nurse how the patient is doing. This essentially social introduction

not only establishes rapport and relieves anxiety but also gives information regarding the ABCs, as in the acutely ill patient. However, always ask yourself whether the ABCs are normal; if doubt exists, then a detailed immediate assessment should be performed. Using the system in this way can help you to avoid simple errors, particularly when you are tired or stressed, and it will also let you get to this point in a few seconds with stable patients.

FULL PATIENT ASSESSMENT

Now that the patient has been immediately stabilised as necessary, the aim is to gather information from a variety of sources that will lead you to a diagnosis of current or potential problems and hence to a plan of action. Your immediate management manoeuvres are not an end in themselves – they simply buy you time to solve the underlying problems.

Chart review

Inspection of the observation and fluid charts, preferably at the end of the bed, together with discussion with the nurse and house surgeon brings to light any recent or outstanding problems and allows a focused clinical assessment to be carried out. Charts, particularly those in the HDU or ICU, may appear to carry an overwhelming amount of data, but this can be handled by systematically noting both **absolute values** and **trends**.

LOGICAL APPROACH TO HDU CHARTS
R Respiratory:
   respiratory rate
   inspired oxygen concentration (FiO_2)
   oxygen saturation (SaO_2)
C Circulation:
   heart rate and rhythm
   blood pressure
   urinary output
   fluid balance
   intravenous lines
   central venous pressure
   pulmonary artery wedge pressure
S Surgical:
   special requirements of this operation
   temperature
   drainage (nature and volume)

It is not possible to give a comprehensive account of management in every potential scenario, but you should consider both general and specific aspects of care. For example, general care includes cardio-respiratory function and fluid balance, whereas following liver surgery one might look specifically for production or drainage of bile, liver function tests (LFTs), albumin, glucose and clotting factor levels.

Check the drug chart to see what new drugs have been given and which of the patient's usual drugs might have been forgotten, as either may be influencing the current clinical findings.

History and systematic examination

The history of the patient's present illness and subsequent treatment is just as important in critical illness as in the rest of clinical practice. However, the impact of comorbid conditions is almost as great, and these are overlooked or underestimated at considerable peril. The patient, their case notes, and nursing and junior staff are the main sources of these types of information; the appropriate source will vary from case to case, depending on your prior knowledge of the patient. On occasion, the patient's family and other professional staff can also supply useful information.

The patient is then examined fully, with particular attention being paid to vital systems, the systems or regions involved by surgery or underlying disease, and potential problems already highlighted. This should follow the standard format, beginning with the hands, and including the neck, chest, abdomen and limbs. Wounds and stomas may also require examination.

The importance of **repeated clinical examination** is often underestimated by inexperienced staff, particularly when it comes to diagnosing incipient problems in silent areas; for example, early signs of atelectasis are much more likely to be detected clinically than radiologically. Equally, we all fail to pick up on signs, and repeated examination, perhaps after 15 minutes, helps to prevent this (see Case history 2.1).

Case history 2.1

You are on the orthopaedic ward at 3am with a trauma case when you are asked to see a 62-year-old patient who is tachycardic (heart rate 110/min) 12 hours after a revision hip arthroplasty. The main ward lights are not on, the patient is distressed and in pain, and the house officer has just started a 500-ml bolus fluid challenge and prescribed more analgesia. Blood pressure is 105/75 mmHg. You think the patient is a little cool peripherally but you are not unduly concerned. You have a cup of coffee and then review the patient again. You realise that despite 500 ml of saline, his perfusion is worse, he is oliguric and he has a distended abdomen. It is now clear to you that the patient may well have continuing surgical bleeding and that more intensive resuscitation and consideration of urgent reoperation are required.

Learning point
Reassessment after a short period of time or following a simple intervention often helps to clarify diagnosis.

Review of available results

Available investigation results should now be reviewed. With emergencies, a great deal of useful data may be available from routine blood tests taken earlier, previous microbiology samples or recent imaging requests, so do not overlook these sources of information. On routine ward rounds, it can be better to wait at the end of the bed for missing results than to resolve to see them later – experience suggests that these tasks slip the memory in the busy routine. Work out a schedule with your junior colleagues that maximises the availability of recent results for your main business ward rounds.

REVIEWING THE AVAILABLE RESULTS
- Biochemistry:
  - profile
  - arterial blood gases
  - glucose level
- Haematology:
  - blood count
  - clotting
  - cross-matched blood available
- Microbiology
- Radiology: review reports or examine films
- Return to charts and review any necessary points

DECIDE AND PLAN: STABLE OR UNSTABLE?

Once you have assessed the patient and the available information, you need to make a decision: is the patient **stable** or **unstable**? A patient whom you are unsure about should be managed as unstable, and you should be very cautious about reassigning as stable patients who have been unstable but who have just responded. Clearly, there are degrees of instability, but training yourself to make this simple decision is important, since it will focus your mind on to one of two very different subsequent approaches.

Stable patients: daily plan

Stable patients have normal signs and are progressing as expected. This will apply to most patients seen on the daily ward round and consequently they will not need the aggressive fluid management used for hypovolaemic patients. A plan must be formulated for such patients. On the ward this will be daily, but in the HDU 12-hourly or more frequent assessment and planning will be needed.

DAILY PLAN

- Investigations:
  - bloods and X-rays
  - specialist opinions
- Removal of drains/tubes
- Oral intake
- Fluid balance and prescription
- Nutrition:
  - requirement
  - route
  - is it being given?
- Physiotherapy: chest and mobility
- Drugs and analgesia
  - therapeutic (eg antibiotics, analgesia)
  - preventive (eg subcutaneous heparin)
  - routine (eg cardiac)
- Move to lower level of care

Ensure that necessary therapeutic drugs, including analgesia, are prescribed. Modify these as the patient recovers. Check that appropriate prophylaxis, particularly against venous thromboembolism, is prescribed. Verify that routine medications are being given, if necessary by an alternative route, and

consider what implications the comorbid condition or its treatment might have for present management or prognosis.

Remember also to speak to the patient to encourage and reassure them. Sum up your plan with clear instructions for your nursing colleagues and junior staff, and make or supervise an entry in the notes.

Plan and sum up.

Unstable patients

If progress is not satisfactory, then further investigation or definitive treatment will be needed. If a cause is already evident from your evaluation, then treatment can be planned directly. Inform your senior and consider whether a higher level of care is needed.

If the patient is unstable or you are unsure:

- Review priorities.
- Is resuscitation required before you begin investigations (often the case) or does it need to be continued simultaneously with proposed investigations (usually the case)?
- How will you achieve that?
- Begin any treatment or support that is obviously necessary at once.
- Does the patient need a higher level of care?

SPECIFIC INVESTIGATIONS

These are carried out as necessary to find out why the patient is unwell and unstable and to let you or others subsequently do something about it. These range from the simple to the very complex. Usually, simple blood tests will have already been sent off during the immediate management phase, but now is the time to check. Likewise, chest X-ray, ECG and various cultures may have already been done or may be needed now.

The safest way to accomplish more complex specific investigations will differ between patients, depending on the test required, the degree of urgency and how sick the patient is. Remember that the radiology department is an **unsafe** place for sick patients unless they have adequate critical care support from medical and nursing staff. The ideal test may have to be forgone in some circumstances, or it may be better to transfer the patient to the ICU for full support before a planned transfer to the radiology department.

Specialist opinions (*eg* cardiology, anaesthesia, ICU) may be required. If you reach an impasse, either of a diagnostic or organisational nature, involve your consultant. Do not give up on a necessary investigation or treatment just because it is difficult to arrange, is at an awkward time or is beyond your expertise. Unstable patients seldom improve spontaneously between 4am and 8am (see Case history 2.2).

Case history 2.2

An elderly patient with known mild heart failure underwent endoscopy and injection treatment of a bleeding duodenal ulcer at 8pm. He became steadily oliguric from 11pm and had two cautious fluid challenges from the house officer. You are asked to see him at 3.35am and note he is not well perfused and is mildly dyspnoeic. You give a further 350 ml saline over 45 minutes without any change in the patient's condition. You are unsure what fluids are required and feel a central line is needed. You are not confident enough to insert one yourself, but your senior cover did not seem too pleased when you spoke to him about another problem earlier. You elect to continue with maintenance fluids until the 8am ward round. By then, the patient is in established renal failure.

Learning points

- Patients do not improve magically between 4am and the 8am ward round.
- Unstable patients require diagnosis and definitive treatment without undue delay.
- Involve senior staff if you do not have the particular skills to deal with a given problem.

Be careful to maintain momentum: on busy wards, multiple small delays at each stage can add up to a lengthy delay in treating the underlying cause, which can result in your previous resuscitation being in vain.

Investigations may take some time, during which you must ask yourself repeatedly:

- Is the present level of physiological support optimal?
- Are we reaching a diagnosis and a definite plan of action?
- Are we doing so quickly enough?

If not, a change of plan is needed.

When you have attended a patient, you must record the event in the case notes. This serves several functions: writing your assessment helps clarify your thoughts, your note tells other staff what happened and lets them gauge the response, you can define clear criteria for further interventions, and the note can be of medicolegal importance.

WRITING YOUR NOTES

- *Name* in capitals, date and time, pager number
- *Assessment:*
  - brief summary of past and present events
  - present clinical features
  - response to any treatment already given (*eg* by house officer)
- *Differential diagnosis*
- *Actions:*
  - resuscitation performed (ABC)
  - investigations and opinions
  - treatment
- *Communications* to relatives, staff, seniors, etc
- *Review:*
  - by you
  - by others
- Parameters for change

DEFINITIVE TREATMENT

The underlying aim of critical care practice is to begin definitive treatment of continuing pathology or complications **as quickly as possible**. All the above steps simply keep the patient alive long enough to get this far, but, unless you treat the real problem adequately, then the patient will deteriorate again and may die. Once the need for intervention is clear to all, the situation may be irretrievable, so speed is of the essence throughout.

Treatment may be medical, surgical, radiological or all three, and co-ordination is important. When the patient is a surgical one, you will need to play a leading role in co-ordinating efforts. Consider where non-operative treatment should best be carried out, by whom and the support that will be necessary. If the patient is transferred, especially if to an area that is unfamiliar with surgical patients (*eg* coronary care unit), then detailed instructions will need to be written in the case notes and frequent review will be necessary to ensure that other surgical aspects of care continue to be delivered, even though the staff are unfamiliar with them.

REASSESSMENT

Finally, once any treatment has been instituted, whether simple fluid therapy or a complex surgical operation, you must reassess the patient to ensure that they have responded to the treatment. The necessary timeframe for doing this will depend on the urgency of the case.

If the patient has not responded adequately, then you need to look all the harder for a different cause to treat. Reassessment is the final step – and, if necessary, the first step in repeating the whole process.

SUMMARY

This system will let you assess all your patients in a similar way. It is the system that many senior surgeons and intensivists have used subconsciously for a long time, but in written form. With practice, the use of a system will let you assess patients without overlooking simple and potentially disastrous things, and it will serve as a framework whereby you can apply your theoretical knowledge to clinical problems.

- Using a structured system to assess critically ill patients reduces serious omissions.
- Identify patients in need of immediate life-saving resuscitation; assess and treat them simultaneously.
- Reach a diagnosis that accounts for clinical deterioration.
- Formulate and institute a plan of definitive treatment.
- Investigations should be selective and should be carried out in a safe environment.
- Repeated clinical assessment is the cornerstone of good practice: it identifies things missed first time around and tells you whether the patient is getting better.
- Inform and involve your senior colleagues at an early stage.
- Consider the level of care necessary at each stage.

Respiratory failure and its prevention in the surgical patient **3**

Objectives

This chapter will help you to:

- Understand the importance of respiratory failure and of its prevention.
- Recognise the patient with respiratory failure and their need for support.
- Provide a management approach to respiratory failure.

- Be familiar with common methods of respiratory support.
- Understand the basic concepts of mechanical ventilation.

INTRODUCTION

The commonest reason for admission to an ICU is to provide airway and ventilatory care to critically ill patients who are unable to maintain their own airway and normal respiratory functions. The **early recognition** of an airway or ventilatory problem together with early appropriate treatment will often **prevent** further deterioration and is the basis of effective resuscitation. Many more patients on surgical wards exhibit signs of respiratory compromise, and their effective management is a sizeable and important part of surgical critical care.

As outlined in Chapter 2, you should look specifically for an airway problem when assessing every patient. Often the patient will respond verbally, but if not you should suspect airway compromise in any obtunded patient. Alteration in the level of consciousness, for whatever reason, will result in loss of airway control, decreased or loss of protective gag and/or laryngeal reflexes, and **increased risk of aspiration** of gastric contents into the lungs. The commonest cause of a decreased level of consciousness in general surgical patients is **hypoxia** and/or **hypercapnia** produced as a result of respiratory failure with failed oxygen uptake alone (type I) or failed oxygen uptake

and carbon dioxide removal together (type II). There are numerous causes of respiratory failure, which may be classified simply into three groups:

- acute fall in functional residual capacity (FRC),
- acute fall in effective lung volume with pulmonary vascular dysfunction, and
- airflow obstruction.

Acute fall in FRC without pulmonary vascular dysfunction may be due to central or myoneural disorders, mechanical failure of chest mechanics after trauma, or other processes that render the lungs stiff and non-compliant. **Acute postoperative atelectasis**, sputum retention, pneumonia, and depression of respiration by analgesic, sedative and neuromuscular blocking drugs fall into this category. Frailty and malnutrition contribute.

An acute fall in FRC with pulmonary vascular dysfunction occurs in conditions such as left ventricular failure, fluid overload, pulmonary hypertension, pulmonary embolism, neurogenic pulmonary oedema and acute respiratory distress syndrome (ARDS).

Airflow obstruction occurs in states with increased lung volume, such as chronic obstructive pulmonary disease and asthma.

Any of these conditions will produce respiratory

failure when the **PaO$_2$ is less than 8 kPa** (the point on the oxygen dissociation curve when rapid desaturation occurs if there is any further fall in PaO$_2$) or if the **PaCO$_2$ rises above 7 kPa**. Although the precise definition of respiratory failure is based on arterial blood gas (ABG) criteria, the initial assessment and management approach should follow the pattern already described.

IMMEDIATE ASSESSMENT AND MANAGEMENT

Remember the ABCs. An unconscious patient with no airway must be resuscitated quickly to prevent hypoxic brain damage. Review airway management in Chapter 2 (see also Table 3.1).

Table 3.1 *Techniques of airway control*

Use simple methods first!

> Chin lift/jaw thrust
> Suction
> Oral Guedel airway
> Nasopharyngeal airway if gag reflex present
> Endotracheal tube
> Surgical airway

Seek anaesthetic help

Always give oxygen

The patient with respiratory failure may be recognised easily if they are:

- dyspnoeic, tachypnoeic or apnoeic;
- unable to speak in complete sentences;
- using accessory muscles of respiration;
- centrally cyanosed;
- sweaty and tachycardic; and/or
- showing a decreased level of consciousness.

Aim to oxygenate the patient using a high-flow oxygen mask of a suitable oxygen delivery percentage if the patient is still breathing. During resuscitation, you should not worry about the possibility of depressing ventilation by giving high concentrations of oxygen to a patient with chronic pulmonary disease who normally requires an hypoxic drive to produce adequate ventilation having become habituated to a high level of arterial carbon dioxide. If the patient needs oxygen that badly, you should give it.

Apply a pulse oximeter. Once the patient has stabilised, the rule is to give the minimum added oxygen to achieve the best oxygenation.

If the patient is apnoeic or has very shallow respiration, then **ventilation** using a bag/valve/mask system is required. This can usually maintain the patient until an anaesthetist arrives. If you do decide to intubate, you should keep in mind the risk of regurgitation and aspiration of stomach contents and apply cricoid pressure before laryngoscopy. If you try to intubate the patient but fail, or if you are unable to ventilate the patient manually, then you are committed to performing a surgical airway by either needle or surgical cricothyroidotomy in order to ensure lifesaving oxygenation and ventilation. The techniques of airway management are covered in the Advanced Trauma Life Support (ATLS®) course supervised by the College and which you are recommended to attend.

FULL PATIENT ASSESSMENT

Chart review

Chart examination may reveal a change in respiratory rate, temperature, pulse rate, blood pressure, colour or amount of sputum produced, or level of consciousness, or may reveal a fall in oxygen saturation or deterioration in ABGs if recorded previously. Fluid balance charts should be examined for signs of fluid overload. A deteriorating trend in any of these physiological variables is an essential diagnostic tool, and accurate charting cannot be overemphasised.

History and systematic examination

You should rapidly review the patient's history in an effort to determine the likely source of respiratory difficulty. The patient may be a known asthmatic or chronic bronchitic or may recently have received a large dose of opiates. If this information is obtainable from the nurses, then you can be examining the patient simultaneously. The examination should initially be clinical, based on simple 'look, listen and feel' techniques described in Chapter 2 and aimed at detecting the physiological changes of developing respiratory failure.

Available results

Full blood count: correction of anaemia will help to improve oxygen delivery to the tissues if the haemoglobin is less than 10 g/dl. Overtransfusion conversely brings the risks of fluid overload and increased blood viscosity. An elevated white cell count may indicate concurrent infection, which may be pneumonic in origin.

The urea and electrolytes may give some indication of fluid and renal status.

ABG sampling is the single most useful blood test in relation to respiratory failure. You should be familiar with the practical skill of sampling and the interpretation of these results. The interpretation of ABGs is outlined at the end of this chapter. Remember to treat the patient as a whole and not to act only on the blood gases in isolation from the clinical findings.

The ECG will provide information regarding the presence or absence of myocardial ischaemia and heart rhythm and rate abnormalities, which may be

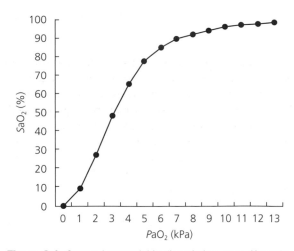

Figure 3.1 *Oxygen haemoglobin dissociation curve. Keep the saturation above 94%*

PULSE OXIMETRY

Pulse oximetry has become a central tool in the monitoring of critically ill surgical patients. You should understand how it works, know its limitations and know how to use it on your patients. It is well recognised that sporadic, brief hypoxic episodes occur in many patients; in some patients, these will result in more prolonged visceral ischaemia.

Understanding the mechanism will make you aware of the limitations. Pulse oximetry works by combining two principles based on light transmission and reception through the tissue. Firstly, the probe detects pulsatile flow plethysmographically. Secondly, it differentiates between oxygenated and reduced haemoglobin by their differing light absorption. Signal processing produces a display of heart rate and arterial oxygen saturation (SaO_2).

Remember that the saturation does not equate to the partial pressure (which is responsible for gas exchange). Recall or revise the oxygen dissociation curve that links these parameters (see Fig. 3.1). Note that an SaO_2 of 90% often equates with a PaO_2 of approximately 8 kPa, so it is advisable to aim to keep the SaO_2 at 95% or more and to set the alarms accordingly.

The pulse oximeter does not detect hypercapnia or acidosis; these require blood gas analysis.

The pulse oximeter is fooled by carboxyhaemoglobin into giving an erroneously high reading. Other factors that impede accurate pulse oximetry include:

- movement, eg shivering, rigors, tremor, agitation,
- peripheral vasoconstriction, eg shock, hypothermia,
- dirty skin,
- profound anaemia,
- diathermy, and
- bright lights.

responsible for the onset or worsening of respiratory failure. Cardiac and respiratory physiological variables are inseparable when it comes to the assessment and treatment of respiratory failure, and further investigations of cardiac function such as echocardiography or cardiac output or index estimations may be appropriate at a higher level of care.

The plain CXR remains a valuable diagnostic tool, but transfer of the unstable patient to the radiology department is **dangerous** and should not delay treatment. Radiographic changes often lag behind the clinical change, and it is important to treat the patient rather than the X-ray. Interpretation of CXRs is covered in the CCrISP course.

Preoperative lung function tests (peak expiratory flow rate, vital capacity, forced expiratory volume in 1s or FEV_1) are useful in predicting the patient at risk, although a patient's ability to climb a flight of stairs in one go or to conduct everyday tasks also provides valuable information.

Infection is the most common cause of respiratory failure, and samples of sputum and blood for culture should be obtained preferably before commencing antibiotic therapy. If the patient is already on antibiotics, then these should be taken before the next dose when antibiotic blood levels are at their lowest. In the intubated patient, sputum samples can be taken by bronchial alveolar lavage (BAL). These give better results since they are uncontaminated by upper-airway flora.

STABLE PATIENT: DAILY MANAGEMENT PLAN

You should consider the adequacy of respiratory function in all patients after major surgery or with critical illness and take steps to prevent problems arising.

Prescribe humidified oxygen therapy by mask at an appropriate concentration. **Monitor** clinical signs (especially respiratory rate), oxygen saturation and ABGs. **Communicate** with nursing staff and ensure that they are aware of the increased frequency of desired observations to be made.

Set parameters beyond which the nursing staff must call for further medical opinion. Commence hourly urine output monitoring if the patient is catheterised and enforce meticulous fluid balance and microbiological surveillance (sputum and blood cultures). The frequency with which early chest problems are encountered cannot be overemphasised; nor can the importance of examining the chest routinely and adopting the simple preventive measures outlined above in a liberal fashion.

Case history 3.1

A 62-year-old woman with mild chronic bronchitis undergoes a right abdominal nephrectomy for carcinoma. You are called to see her on the evening of the second postoperative day because she has become difficult to rouse. Immediate assessment shows her to be obtunded and failing to maintain her airway adequately. She is cyanosed but well perfused.

You clear the airway with suction and a chin lift. She tolerates an oropharyngeal airway and you administer high-flow oxygen, relieving the cyanosis. Over the next few minutes, her conscious level improves and the airway can be removed.

You review her in detail and find that her epidural is working only poorly, that no oxygen therapy has been given for six hours and that she has not seen the physiotherapist today. She has poor air entry bilaterally, particularly at the right base. Blood gases now show a mild respiratory acidosis and a $PaCO_2$ just above the upper limit of normal.

The patient is transferred to the HDU and a pulse oximeter attached. You prescribe humidified oxygen to maintain her saturation above 95% and start regular nebulised salbutamol as she uses salbutamol as necessary at home. A chest radiograph (CXR) is requested (see Fig. 3.2). You arrange for immediate review by the on-call physiotherapist and the pain

team. The physiotherapist obtains a sputum sample for culture, but, because this looks clear and the patient has a normal white cell count, you elect not to start antibiotics at present.

You review the patient one hour later and confirm that her improved analgesia has allowed her to increase her air entry and clearance of secretions and thereby her oxygenation. Her gases have improved. You discuss her case with the HDU nurse and agree the necessary frequency of observations and parameters of saturation, respiratory rate and pain score that would necessitate further urgent medical review. You plan to review the patient in any event at 8am to discuss her with (and feedback to) her own team.

Learning points
- Predict the patients at risk and establish the correct level of care from the outset.
- Regular nursing observations and medical review: once daily is not enough in some cases.
- Use preventive techniques liberally, including chest physiotherapy, nebulised saline, monitored humidified oxygen, adequate analgesia and sputum culture.

PREVENTING RESPIRATORY DETERIORATION FOLLOWING SURGERY
- Examine and assess.
- Chest physiotherapy.
- Nebulised saline.
- Humidified oxygen, titrated dose.
- Adequate analgesia.
- Sputum culture.
- Reassess.

PRACTICAL SKILL: INTERPRETING CHEST X-RAYS

Objectives
- To learn a system for examining chest X-rays in the critically ill.
- To be aware of the complementary information provided by clinical and radiographic examination.

The CXR is one of the most frequently ordered investigations in the management of critically ill patients. In many cases, abnormal signs will be picked up earlier on clinical examination, as radiographic appearances tend to lag behind the clinical findings. The CXR offers valuable confirmatory and complementary diagnostic evidence (or reassurance). The aim here is not to list exhaustively the clinical scenarios and diagnoses where it may be of help, but rather to teach a system of reading a CXR.

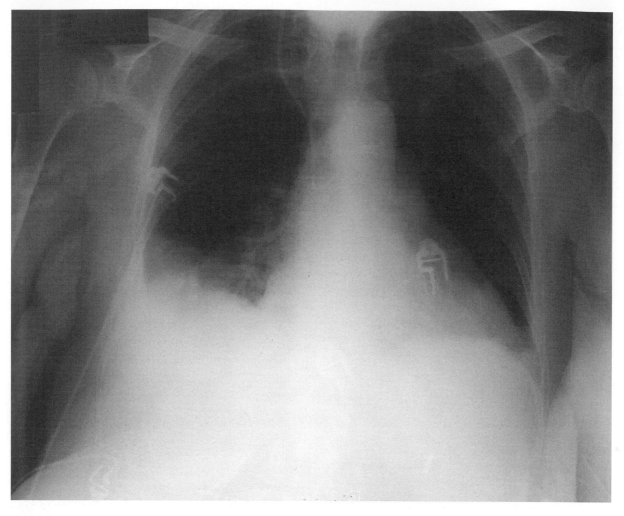

Figure 3.2 *CXR. Confirmed to be a recent film of the patient in Case history 2.1. Obvious abnormalities include shadowing right base, CVP line and ECG leads. Detailed assessment shows blunting of left costophrenic angle, no pneumothorax from CVP line, and ?cardiomegaly (but anteroposterior (AP) film). Conclude no features to suggest different pathology to marked atelectasis*

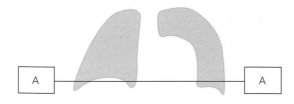

Figure 3.3 *Draw a line across the lower part of the CXR to include the costophrenic angle as shown (A–A). The line passes through the structures to be examined in order*

Table 3.2 *Systematic assessment of the CXR*

Soft tissues	Surgical emphysema, tubes, foreign bodies
Bones	Fractures, deformity
Pleura	Pneumo/haemothorax
Lung parenchyma	Volume, clear?
Costophrenic angles	Clear?
Diaphragms	?Air beneath, ?suggestion of abdominal problems
Mediastinum	Width and position of components, tubes and lines

Use a routine when looking at CXRs, otherwise you may miss other pathology.

The most useful chest view for assessing the heart is a straight, erect posteroanterior (PA), taken at full inspiration. This type of X-ray is more likely to give a true indication of heart size than the anteroposterior (AP). Unfortunately, often only the portable AP films are available, where artefactual cardiomegaly may be seen. Be aware of which type you are looking at and remember to check the name, date, time and side. Compare with previous films.

Your routine should be (see also Table 3.2):

- Note the overall shape of the chest and obvious abnormalities.
- Use a system to assess the CXR fully. One system is the line method (see Fig. 3.3).
- Note soft-tissue abnormalities, such as air (surgical emphysema), foreign bodies or disruption of contours.
- The bony structures are remembered by the Collegiate mnemonic RCS's: ribs, clavicles, scapulae, sternum.
- Do the pulmonary markings extend to the chest wall? Is there pneumothorax or haemothorax? Trace around the edge of the pleural cavity to avoid missing a small pneumothorax. Is the volume of parenchyma increased (chronic obstructive airways disease (COAD), lots of ribs visible) or reduced (poor respiratory effort, abdominal distension)?
- Examine the CXR from near and far, looking at the lung fields for opacities. The size and distribution of the pulmonary vessels may occasionally show evidence of pulmonary embolism, but usually only if the embolus is large.
- Double-check the costophrenic angles for fluid (erect film?).
- Is there air beneath the diaphragm (erect film) or any obvious intra-abdominal abnormality to investigate specifically (eg distended bowel)?
- Note tracheal position and heart size. Trace around the mediastinum and check the location of any tubes or lines. The width of the mediastinum should be noted but may be unreliable. Combined with a history suggestive of aortic aneurysm or trauma, a second opinion should be sought immediately.

Air bronchogram

A bronchus is not normally visible if surrounded by normal aerated lung, since both are equally radio-opaque. Anything that causes the normal lung tissue to lose its aerated property will produce a difference in opaqueness, and the bronchus, provided it still contains air, will be visible. Thus, the presence of an air bronchogram suggests oedema, infection or other infiltrates in the surrounding lung tissue.

Kerley B lines

These are horizontal lines that meet the pleural surface at right angles. They tend to be about 1–2 cm long and 1–2 mm thick. They are caused by increased fluid or tissue within the intralobular septa.

Bronchitis and emphysema

Bronchitis and emphysema can be present with few or no CXR abnormalities. What may be present is increased lucency of the lung and regional or general loss of vascularity in the peripheral lung fields. The lung fields are increased in size.

Pleural effusion

A small effusion may produce only a blunting of the costophrenic angle. A large effusion will produce evidence of lung compression, usually respiratory problems, and the mediastinum may be displaced to the opposite side and the diaphragm flattened on that side. It is important to be aware that, on an X-ray taken with the patient supine, an effusion may show only as a faint diffuse opacity spread over the lung field. This is because the fluid is spread thinly over a wide area. Repeat the X-ray with the patient having been sat up for 15 minutes, or obtain an ultrasound scan. An effusion due to cardiac disorder tends to be bilateral.

Consolidation

Consolidation will not produce a mediastinal shift unless there is significant collapse, when the mediastinum will be drawn over to the side of the lesion.

Pericardial effusion

There are many reasons for an enlarged cardiac silhouette, which can be apparent (see Table 3.3) or pathological. The most common pathological reasons include ventricular hypertrophy, pericardial effusion and ventricular aneurysm. An effusion may produce an outline that is globular in appearance, but hypertrophy of the left ventricle can do the same. Left atrial enlargement can produce a straightening of the left cardiac border. A significant pericardial effusion is likely to produce evidence of tamponade, with poor cardiac function and a raised central venous pressure. If in doubt, ultrasound will confirm the diagnosis.

Cardiac failure

Cardiac failure may give rise to a variety of signs, including upper lobe blood diversion, cardiomegaly, pleural effusions, Kerley B lines and parenchymal shadowing (diffuse or hilar 'bat's wing').

Table 3.3 *Causes of apparent cardiomegaly*
Chamber enlargement – athletes
Technical (AP view)
High diaphragm
Cardiac fat pads
Skeletal deformity

MANAGEMENT OF RESPIRATORY FAILURE AND COMPROMISE

The treatment plan for managing respiratory failure follows a stepwise increase/decrease in support, depending on its severity (see Fig. 3.4). During initiation of treatment, you start at the left of the scale and progress to the right, as determined by your assessment of the patient's response.

Only conventional mask oxygen therapy is possible on the majority of surgical wards. Fixed-delivery oxygen masks are available up to an inspired oxygen concentration of 60% or a fractional inspired oxygen concentration (FiO_2) of 0.6%. All oxygen delivery systems should be **humidified**, otherwise the dry, cold gas may contribute towards thickening of the patient's secretions and promote sputum retention. Nebulised 0.9% saline (plus bronchodilators if indicated) and regular treatment from a respiratory physiotherapist may prevent worsening of incipient respiratory failure if used early.

The response of the patient is assessed according to the improvement of clinical status, oxygen saturation and ABG analyses. If the patient's condition does not improve with increased inspired oxygen

concentration up to 60%, then you have a very unstable patient and further diagnosis and definitive treatment are required. This will involve expert help and the safe transfer of the patient to a higher level of care.

Even if the patient responds to supplemental oxygen therapy and the ABGs improve, you must remember that oxygen is only **one aspect** of treatment: you must treat the underlying cause of the respiratory failure.

Treating the cause of respiratory failure or compromise

Supportive and definitive treatments are needed. Use appropriate antibiotics, physiotherapy, diuretics, bronchodilators and cardiac or other drugs, as necessary. Basal signs may indicate continuing abdominal pathology (*eg* subphrenic abscess). Systemic factors influence respiratory function (*eg* mobility, nutrition); it is important to treat these as well.

Review the patient's requirement for and response to **analgesia**; either too little or too much can be a factor in preventing adequate clearance of secretions by inhibiting coughing and by limiting their tolerance of physiotherapy. Where sputum clearance is the primary problem, a mini-tracheostomy should be considered. Do not assume that confusion or a depressed level of consciousness is due to the effects of opiate analgesia. Hypoxia may cause an acute confusional state, and hypercapnia may lead to obtundation.

Reassessment

Detect failure of improvement or deterioration: persisting or worsening signs and symptoms of respiratory failure necessitate further immediate management and safe transfer to a higher level of care.

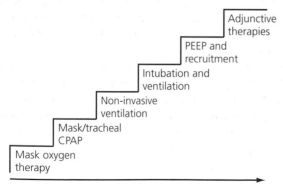

Figure 3.4 *Treatment plan for managing respiratory failure. CPAP, continuous positive airway pressure; PEEP, positive end expiratory pressure*

Detecting failure of simple oxygen therapy

It is essential to be alert to this situation, as it is common, can be rapidly fatal and requires a prompt change in management. Failure of mask oxygen therapy at high FiO_2 may be indicated by:

- increasing **respiratory rate**;
- increasing **distress**, dyspnoea, exhaustion, sweating and confusion;
- oxygen saturation of 80% or less (this may be a late sign);
- PaO_2 less than 8 kPa; and/or
- $PaCO_2$ greater than 7 kPa.

The clinical signs and blood gas analysis are the most important. Tachypnoeic patients tire and arrest suddenly. You must intervene **before** this stage by acting on early symptoms and signs, particularly tachypnoea. Transfer the patient to a higher level of care for further therapy to improve gas exchange. An arterial line should be inserted if frequent blood gas analysis is to be performed. Anticipate problems in patients with severe chronic lung disease (*eg* vital capacity less than 15 ml/kg or FEV_1 less than 10 ml/kg) and monitor closely.

Case history 3.2

The 62-year-old woman seen in Case history 3.1 with chronic bronchitis and right abdominal nephrectomy responded well initially to the measures you instituted.

However, it is now four days postoperative, and this morning she was noted to be tachypnoeic and pyrexial, with reduced air entry, bronchial breathing and dullness to percussion at the right lung base. Her FiO_2 was increased to 0.8 in order to maintain SaO_2 above 97%. The physiotherapist obtained a sample of foul sputum for culture, and ceftriaxone 1 g was prescribed for pneumonia. A CXR showed typical localised changes at the right base.

It is now 7pm and the HDU nurse has called you because the patient is again tachypnoeic and hypoxic despite the therapy described above. Chest signs are unchanged but the patient is noticeably sweaty and starting to look tired. She is not in pain and on detailed review there does not seem to be anything else you can do to improve matters. Recent blood gases show that the PCO_2 has risen from 4 kPa to 7.3 kPa over the last 10 hours.

The HDU nurse is experienced and is worried that the patient might tire and arrest suddenly. You accept her advice and ask for an urgent ICU review. The ICU consultant is pleased that you called at this stage. Continuous positive airway pressure (CPAP) on the HDU is considered, but the patient is hypercapnic and it is decided to take her to the ICU for intubation and ventilation.

Learning points

- Use your routine ward rounds to monitor progress systematically, but reassess and hand over patients who are not right at the end of the routine day.
- Detect patients who are failing to respond or deteriorating despite reasonable therapy and refer promptly.
- Clinical signs (eg tiredness and sweating) are also important in detecting the patient at risk of respiratory failure and arrest.

Continuous positive airway pressure

If the primary problem is type I respiratory failure (hypoxia with normal CO_2), then CPAP by mask may help. A tight-fitting facemask with a range of expiratory valves that do not open until a pressure of $2.5–10 \, cmH_2O$ is applied to the patient with a high-flow source of oxygen-enriched air. As the patient expires against the resistance of the valve, or as gas flows into the patient during inspiration, the pressure in the airways should not drop below the pressure indicated on the valve. This opens any alveoli that may be closed and prevents their collapse on expiration. This recruitment of under-ventilated alveoli increases FRC, decreases intra-pulmonary shunt and may improve oxygenation. The masks are uncomfortable to wear, may cause nasal pressure sores and, if air-swallowing occurs, may result in gastric dilation and regurgitation. Some patients unable to tolerate a full facemask may tolerate a nasal mask, but the patient must keep the mouth closed to prevent loss of pressure. CPAP may also be connected directly via a T-piece to a pre-existing tracheostomy tube. The patient must have a reasonable respiratory rate and tidal volume, be in control of their own airway and be able to co-operate. Patients who fail to tolerate CPAP are recognised by refractory hypoxaemia, increasing respiratory rate and progressively smaller tidal volumes, with subsequent CO_2 retention.

Non-invasive ventilation by mask

If type II respiratory failure (CO_2 retention) develops, non-invasive ventilatory support should be considered. In this mode of respiratory support, the level of CPAP is alternated between a high and a low level at a fixed frequency. This may be termed bilevel or BiPAP mask ventilation. The higher CPAP level is set at around $20\,cmH_2O$ at inspiration and the lower level at $5\,cmH_2O$ during expiration. The pressure difference between the two levels will generate gas flow into the lungs during inspiration. The BiPAP machine detects patient inspiration by the initial drop in airway pressure that occurs on inspiration and automatically raises the pressure to the top pressure set on the machine and changes to the lower level on expiration. The tidal volume delivered is determined by the lung compliance, the duration of inspiration and the driving pressure. This method of respiratory support may pre-empt the requirement for intubation and ventilation. This type of ventilation may be used on respiratory HDUs or surgical HDUs, provided staff are trained in its use. It is not effective in all patients, and careful selection is required. It is not appropriate for patients who are cardiovascularly unstable, have decreased level of consciousness, have a severe metabolic acidosis or have poor respiratory rates. The patient must be in control of their own airway and be able to co-operate. Patients who fail to tolerate mask ventilation are recognised by refractory hypoxaemia, increasing respiratory rate and progressively smaller tidal volumes, with worsening CO_2 retention. In general terms, if the patient's CO_2 has not improved within 30 minutes, then mask ventilation is unlikely to succeed.

Controlled mechanical ventilation

This form of ventilation requires admission to the ICU because intubation is required. Intubation provides a definitive airway and is always required for safe positive-pressure ventilation in patients where aspiration of gastric contents into the lungs is a risk. Intubation and ventilation allow oxygen concentrations of up to 100%, and the volume of each breath (tidal volume, V_T) and respiratory rate or frequency (f) may be adjusted to suit the patient's needs. The minute volume (MV; also termed minute ventilation) is calculated from $V_T \times f$ and may be varied by altering either the frequency or the tidal volume. The greater the minute volume, the greater the removal of carbon dioxide. Too large a tidal volume may damage the lung; in general, 6–8 ml/kg body weight is used. This form of ventilation requires a fully sedated patient to tolerate the presence of the tracheal tube

and the compulsory positive pressure breaths from the ventilator. This mode of ventilation allows the patient to play no part in breathing and is used rarely. Most commonly, a synchronised intermittent mandatory ventilation (SIMV) mode is used to try to preserve some of the patient's respiratory muscle activity.

Lung compliance, tidal volume and how fast the tidal volume is 'pushed' into the patient determine the pressure reached within the airways at the end of each breath from the ventilator. This peak airway pressure has adverse consequences. The intrathoracic pressure is always positive on inspiration during ventilation. This causes decreased venous return and a fall in cardiac output, which may be very severe if the patient is hypovolaemic. Positive end expiratory pressure (PEEP) makes this effect even worse. PEEP is used to recruit underventilated alveoli and to prevent others from collapsing by ensuring that, at the end of expiration, the airway pressure does not fall to zero (relative to atmospheric pressure). High values of peak airway pressure and PEEP predispose to barotrauma, which can result in rapid formation of a tension pneumothorax. Also, prophylactic drainage of a simple pneumothorax before positive-pressure ventilation prevents it expanding and 'tensioning'.

High pressures plus high oxygen concentrations may also promote the toxic effects of oxygen; consequently, concentrations of oxygen of more than 80% are used rarely, and then only for the shortest possible time. Peak airway pressures of greater than $35\,cmH_2O$ and the use of large tidal volumes cause overdistension of alveoli and damage to vascular endothelial tight junctions. This process of volutrauma promotes alveolar and vascular damage, resulting in fluid leak and worsening of lung compliance, which in turn predisposes to even higher airway pressures.

Pressure-limited or pressure-controlled ventilation is used to prevent airway pressures exceeding $35\,cmH_2O$, which, together with a maximum tidal volume of 8 ml/kg, aims to prevent ventilator-induced lung injury. When lung compliance is so poor that airway pressures exceed $35\,cmH_2O$, tidal volumes may be so small that normal carbon dioxide removal is not possible. Rather than increase the tidal volume beyond safe levels, the $PaCO_2$ is left high (permissive hypercapnia) in order to minimise lung damage. This is known as a lung-protective ventilatory strategy. It must be combined with lung-recruitment strategies such as PEEP, occasional large tidal breaths, regular physiotherapy, suction and turning the patient to prevent alveolar collapse. Lung recruitment aims to open as many poorly compliant alveoli as possible and to prevent their collapse and consolidation. CXR, ultrasonography or fibre-optic bronchoscopy should be used to identify any lung collapse or compression amenable to treatment. This could include lobar collapse requiring bronchoscopic reinflation, pleural effusions or undiagnosed pneumothoraces.

Normally, the ventilator is set to provide less time for inspiration than expiration. If the lungs are very poorly compliant and 'stiff', then the inspiratory time may be increased to be equal to or even longer than the expiratory time. This process is known as adjusting the inspiratory to expiratory (I:E) ratio. The I:E ratio may thus be normal (1:2 or 1:3), equal (1:1) or inverse (2:1). Applying a limited pressure for a prolonged period of time aims to improve gas exchange by opening the poorly compliant alveoli, holding them open for as long as possible to maximise gas exchange at pressures that will not cause barotrauma or volutrauma or decrease cardiac output.

A patient on pressure-controlled inverse ratio ventilation (PCIRV), a high FiO_2 of more than 0.8, PEEP greater than $10 \, cmH_2O$ and permissive hypercapnia who fails to achieve oxygen saturation of greater than 85% is very likely to die. Death will occur from multiple organ failure as tissue oxygen delivery fails to meet demand. At this point, the use of an FiO_2 of 1.0 is justified and other adjuncts to ventilation may be considered. The most commonly used adjunct is to turn the patient from the supine to the prone position. Redistribution of blood flow to the less consolidated or collapsed, more easily ventilated anterior portions of the lung may result in improved oxygenation. Other methods to improve oxygenation include the use of inhaled pulmonary vasodilators such as nitric oxide or epoprostenol (prostacyclin). Finally, extracorporeal life support (ECLS) with veno-venous cardiopulmonary bypass could be considered. None of these adjuncts to oxygenation has been shown in prospective randomised controlled trials in adults to improve survival: survival depends on adequate treatment of the underlying cause of organ failure.

Weaning from ventilatory support

Whatever the method of mechanical ventilatory support used, if treatment of the underlying cause of respiratory failure has been successful, then the patient must be 'weaned' from the ventilator, ie returned to spontaneous respiration, in a safe, controlled manner. As soon as the patient is able to participate in ventilation, they should be encouraged to do so, since prolonged ventilation will lead to atrophy of the respiratory muscles.

In general, it is unwise to attempt weaning until:

- the original cause of respiratory failure has been treated successfully;
- sedative drugs have been reduced to a level where they will not depress respiration;
- a low inspired oxygen concentration (40%) maintains a normal PaO_2;
- CO_2 elimination is no longer a problem;
- sputum production is minimal;
- nutritional status, minerals and trace elements are normal;
- neuromuscular function of the diaphragm and intercostals is adequate;
- the patient is reasonably co-operative.

Various modes of ventilation are available, which allow a gradually increasing amount of breathing to be performed by the patient as their condition improves. The transition from pressure-controlled ventilation (PCV) to other modes allowing some patient input to ventilation is not an exact science, and none of the objective measurements of respiratory function has found widespread acceptance as a predictor of successful weaning. The step-down modes from PCV are numerous, but the most commonly used are SIMV, assisted spontaneous breathing (ASB) and pressure-support ventilation (PSV). Often, ASB and PSV are used in conjunction with the other modes.

As an alternative to these gradual reductions in the mechanical component of ventilation, a simple T-piece may be used for periods of time, allowing the patient to do all the breathing before being put back on mechanical ventilation when they show objective signs of diminished respiratory effort. The periods of time spent breathing spontaneously are increased until extubation is possible. In the majority of critical care units, a combined approach is used, with PCV, then SIMV, ASB/PSV, CPAP, T-piece and finally extubation. Patients may fail extubation as a result of poor airway control, laryngeal oedema, poor cough, sputum retention or simple fatigue.

Where the requirement for ventilation is

prolonged, a tracheostomy is often performed to prevent the adverse effects of prolonged tracheal intubation and to facilitate weaning by allowing decreased sedation and ease of reventilation. The timing of elective tracheostomy is controversial, and there is no universally accepted practice. Tracheostomy on the critical care unit is performed frequently using dilational, percutaneous methods rather than the open surgical technique. The track takes up to seven days to form, and these tubes should not be replaced earlier unless absolutely necessary. After seven days, the tubes should be replaced with tubes that contain an inner cannula, which can be removed for cleaning. Regular suction and humidification will help to prevent obstruction. If the tracheostomy tube occludes completely, let down the cuff and remove and replace it. Routine tracheostomy care will be discussed during the CCrISP course.

WARD MANAGEMENT OF PATIENTS WITH A TRACHEOSTOMY

The management of tracheostomy on the wards is straightforward, provided simple principles are followed:

- Determine when and what type of tracheostomy the patient received.
- Replace with a variety with a removable inner tube to facilitate cleaning as soon as possible.
- If you do not know how to replace/change the tube, always ask for help.
- Humidification and regular suction are essential.
- Consider removal of tracheostomy only when the initial indication for its presence has been resolved.
- Assess swallowing/laryngeal competence before cuff deflation; a formal assessment by speech and language therapists is useful.
- Deflate cuff after ensuring the patient's pharynx is empty.
- If the patient can cough, expectorate, phonate and protect their airway with the cuff deflated, then the prospects for decannulation are good. Cap the tube to assess this only **after** cuff deflation.
- The use of specialised tracheostomy tubes requires input from ear, nose and throat (ENT) or ICU colleagues.
- After decannulation, dress and occlude the stoma, eg with sterile gauze covered with 'sleek'.
- Always remember that tracheostomy tubes can block: removal may be necessary. If the patient cannot breathe spontaneously via the stoma, then establish an airway by other means. Call for help!

DISCHARGE FROM ICU

The period following ICU discharge is a critical one. Particularly when transfer occurs to a general ward (*ie* without a stopover in an HDU), the patient has to adapt to a reduced level of care in terms of nursing, physiotherapy and monitoring. A discharge summary and suggested treatment plan will usually accompany the patient as they leave the ICU, but it is important that this is understood by the ward staff and is implemented directly. Experience shows that this does not happen automatically. This period of care exemplifies the importance of good personal communication and organisation: communication between ICU and surgical staff and between surgical and ward staff of clear written instructions and repeated assessment of the patient. Apart from clinical reassessment, ensure that medications have been changed to ward format and started, arrange out-of-hours physiotherapy as needed, check the oxygen concentration needed and ensure that any monitoring (*eg* pulse oximetry) is available on the ward. Speak to the on-call team and ask them to formally review the patient during the evening. If the patient deteriorates, contact the ICU staff at an early stage, but usually attention to the details of care and **ensuring** they actually happen will prevent this.

SUMMARY

- Assess respiratory function in all ward patients who have undergone major surgery and use simple measures liberally to **prevent** major respiratory compromise.
- Routine assessment is predominantly clinical and aims to identify the patient who is deteriorating.
- Use the system of assessment to identify clinically those patients with respiratory failure.
- Instigate the level of treatment appropriate to the severity of failure.
- Treat the cause of the failure as well as hypoxia/hypercapnia.
- Reassess clinical signs, oximetry and, most importantly, ABGs.
- Organise safe transfer to a higher level of care for those who do not respond.

ARTERIAL BLOOD GASES AND ACID–BASE BALANCE

ABG measurements are an important adjunct in the management of critically ill surgical patients. They provide an assessment of oxygenation, carbon dioxide excretion and acid–base balance and thus give a measurement of respiratory, renal and cardiovascular function, including tissue perfusion.

Samples for ABGs are obtained by arterial puncture or from an in-dwelling arterial line (a-line). Both techniques can damage arteries (with consequences of distal ischaemia or mycotic aneurysm), but modestly repeated puncture is the less hazardous method. Techniques and risks of a-line placement are covered in Chapter 6 and the CCrISP practical sessions. Punctures are usually made in the radial artery at the wrist, and the demonstration of a patent ulnar artery (Allen's test) provides reassurance that ischaemic damage is unlikely. An oblique angle of entry improves the chance of successful sampling.

PaO_2 complements SaO_2 and is a better indicator of the pressure driving oxygen into the tissues. Whatever other ABG values show, hypoxia should be treated with oxygen therapy. Normal PaO_2 depends on FiO_2. Remember that, as the FiO_2 increases towards 1.0, so the PaO_2 should increase: a PaO_2 of 100 mmHg indicates good oxygenating ability for an individual breathing air (FiO_2 0.21) but not for a patient on high-flow oxygen.

Pulse oximetry does not measure CO_2 but blood gases do. Acute hypercapnia needs increased ventilation (see below).

Acid–base balance

The concentration of hydrogen ions within the body is normally controlled tightly at 40 nmol/l, which is 7.42 pH units. $pH = -\log_{10} [H^+]$.

Over 1000 mmol of hydrogen ions is produced per day, primarily as a result of the production of carbon dioxide. This is excreted by the action of the lung and is dependent upon the minute ventilation as controlled by chemoreceptors in the medulla.

There is also a smaller quantity of hydrogen ions produced as non-volatile acid (phosphates, sulphates, etc) products of metabolism of non-carbohydrate substrate. This amounts to approximately 1 mmol $H^+/kg/24$ h and must be excreted by the distal nephron.

There are therefore two control mechanisms maintaining hydrogen ion homeostasis: respiratory and renal. The **respiratory** mechanism is a rapid-response system that requires normal central nervous system function (central pH chemoreceptors) and lung function to allow carbon dioxide to be transferred from pulmonary venous blood to alveolar gas and excreted in expired gas. Any dysfunction of the mechanics or control of respiration will cause retention of CO_2 and a rise in hydrogen ions – respiratory acidosis – or overexcretion and a fall in hydrogen ions – respiratory alkalosis.

The **renal** mechanism is a slower-responding system that depends upon the excretion of hydrogen ions in the urine by the distal nephron. Conditions that impair renal function and in particular distal nephron function, *eg* obstructive uropathy and circulating volume depletion, will prevent non-volatile hydrogen ion excretion, resulting in a metabolic acidosis.

Proteins are the primary buffer of retained hydrogen ions, but because of the importance of the carbon dioxide/bicarbonate system in the elimination of hydrogen ions, the acid–base status of the body is best reflected by the measurement of carbon dioxide tension and bicarbonate level in the blood. This measures both the volatile and non-volatile arms of the system:

$$H^+ + HCO_3^- \leftrightharpoons H_2CO_3 \leftrightharpoons H_2O + CO_2$$

Non-volatile	Volatile
(Renal)	(Respiratory)

Respiratory acidosis

The retention of carbon dioxide will cause a rise of H^+ by driving the above equation to the left. The kidney will respond slowly over 48 hours to compensate by increasing H^+ excretion in the distal nephron, thus returning H^+ concentration towards, but not completely to, normal.

Metabolic acidosis

The inability of the kidney to excrete non-volatile hydrogen ions or a sudden increase in non-volatile acid load (such as in sepsis) will drive the equation to the right. Respiratory function will respond rapidly by increasing minute volume, reducing CO_2 and causing hydrogen ions to return towards normal.

Respiratory alkalosis

Respiratory alkalosis is caused by the minute ventilation being higher than that required to maintain the PCO_2 appropriate for a hydrogen ion concentration of 40 nmol/l. The PCO_2 is driven down and the hydrogen ion concentration falls (pH rises). This is usually caused by an increased central respiratory drive, commonly caused by fever, hepatic disease, aspirin toxicity or central nervous system dysfunction.

Metabolic alkalosis

Metabolic alkalosis is found when the level of bicarbonate in the blood is increased due either to abnormal retention of (chloride depletion due to loop diuretics) or administration of bicarbonate or to the loss of non-volatile acid from the body (gastric outlet obstruction or chronic nasogastric aspiration).

Knowing the hydrogen ion concentration/pH, PCO_2 and bicarbonate allows the acid–base status to be determined and the type of abnormality and degree of compensation to be estimated. The bicarbonate value most helpful for this is the standardised bicarbonate, which corrects the measured bicarbonate to the value that would be present if the PCO_2 was normal (40 mmHg or 5.4 kPa). The non-volatile acid–base state is also summarised by the calculated base excess, which gives a value of the difference between the standardised bicarbonate and the normal value of 24 mmol/l.

MANAGEMENT OF ACID–BASE DISTURBANCE

The primary aim must be the determination of the type of acidosis/alkalosis and thereafter its cause. Clearly, a primary respiratory problem will direct attention to the respiratory and central nervous systems and a metabolic problem to the source of increased non-volatile hydrogen ions or impairment of renal function.

Metabolic acidosis

- Impaired tissue perfusion: deal with cause, improve circulation/perfusion.
- Renal failure: deal with cause, bicarbonate, renal replacement therapy.
- Hepatic failure: ?transplantation.

Respiratory acidosis

- Head or spinal injury: ventilation.
- Drug overdose: antidote (*eg* naloxone) and/or ventilation if indicated.
- Chest wall deformity or injury: ventilation if indicated.
- Myopathy or peripheral neuropathy: ventilation if indicated.
- Pulmonary disease: treat disease and ventilation if indicated.
- Massive pulmonary embolus: re-establish perfusion of ventilated lung.

The method of correction of any abnormality will obviously vary with the cause and also with the degree of chronic compensation. Administration of bicarbonate or artificial ventilation must be controlled by the measurement of the change in hydrogen ion concentration in order not to overcorrect and cause problems such as seizures or tetany by too rapid a fall in hydrogen ion concentration.

SUMMARY

- pH indicates whether there is acidosis or alkalosis.
- Base excess indicates whether acidosis is metabolic (negative base excess) or respiratory.
- Low PaO_2 indicates the presence of hypoxia.
- High $PaCO_2$ and acidosis (plus high HCO_3^- and positive base excess) indicate respiratory acidosis.

Objectives

This chapter will help you to:

- Assess your patient to see if their cardiovascular system (CVS) is functioning adequately.
- Determine whether the problem is primarily cardiovascular in origin.
- Determine the most likely underlying pathology.
- Decide where and how this should be treated appropriately.
- Initiate safe and appropriate management of common cardiac pathologies.

Chapters 4, 5 and 6 deal with aspects of cardiovascular disorders, shock and monitoring and should be considered together. This first chapter will introduce a basic pattern of thinking that will enable an impending cardiovascular problem to be detected early. Preventive measures, simple treatments or referral to a specialist unit can then be initiated. This chapter will focus on clinical assessment and the diagnosis and management of cardiac disorders. Management and treatment of shock are dealt with separately in Chapter 5.

Disorders of the CVS are very common in the sick surgical patient. They can be due to associated medical **comorbidity** or they can arise as **complications** following surgical procedures. Despite the presence of an intact airway and adequate ventilation, any problem causing decreased efficiency of the CVS can result in inadequate delivery of oxygen to the tissues for their metabolic needs, which will initiate a cascade of adverse events that will lead to the development of organ failure. The range of pathologies that cause CVS disturbance is immense, including too little circulating volume, too much volume, primary 'pump' problems, too high an afterload and too low an afterload. While organ failure may be obvious, it often presents initially as a collection of symptoms that occur in the presence of apparently 'normal' or slightly deranged pulse rates and blood pressure. Early recognition of an impending disaster and initiation of treatment will increase your patient's chances of survival and help to prevent further complications, eg renal failure as a result of hypotension and reduced renal perfusion. **Prediction and prevention** are vital.

For these reasons, the approach to the examination of the CVS must be systematic, accurately documented and repeated. The effect of any intervention undertaken (eg fluid administration) must be reassessed to ensure its efficacy and durability.

PATIENT ASSESSMENT AND MANAGEMENT

Immediate assessment and resuscitation

In order to establish that the patient does not need immediate lifesaving resuscitation, you need to make your immediate assessment of the patient based on the ABCs, so check (and correct) the ABCs as necessary. Keep an open mind; do not try to make the findings fit any preconceived diagnosis. Common things are common, and hypovolaemia due to haemorrhage or unreplaced fluid losses should be considered the primary cause of CVS dysfunction in the surgical patient until proved otherwise. Thereafter, sepsis, cardiac dysfunction and pulmonary embolism are the most common problems.

Dyspnoea makes a cardiac and/or respiratory cause more likely. Breathing and the CVS are inextricably linked: a disorder of the respiratory system (*eg* tension pneumothorax) may produce CVS signs, and a CVS disorder (*eg* left ventricular failure) may produce respiratory signs.

All other organ systems are dependent on the viability of the circulation. This is particularly true of the renal and the central nervous systems, and the integrity of these end organs can give valuable information about the function of the CVS. If the patient is obtunded or too confused to respond coherently, then cerebral hypoperfusion or hypoxia is likely and prompt action will be needed.

Life-threatening CVS disorders are recognised if you:

- *look* for pallor, poor peripheral perfusion, underfilled or overfilled veins, obvious blood loss from wounds, drains or stomas, swelling of soft tissues or other evidence of concealed haemorrhage into chest, abdomen or pelvis, and ankle or sacral oedema;
- *listen* to the patient: confusion might be due to poor cerebral perfusion; if they say they feel faint on sitting up or are thirsty, consider hypovolaemia. A complaint of breathlessness on lying flat may point to fluid overload. Complaints of chest pain, breathlessness and feeling feverish or cold are all helpful in determining underlying pathology and should not be ignored. Listen to the chest and heart; and

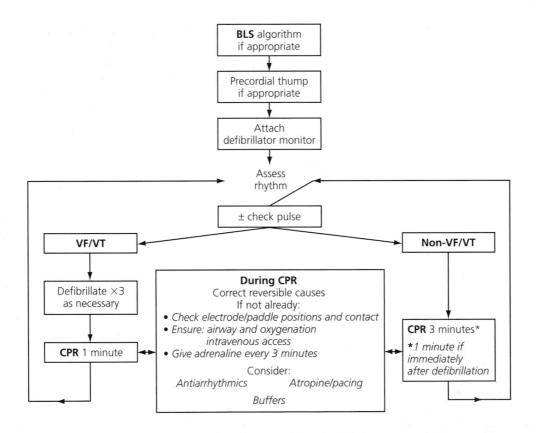

Figure 4.1 *Resuscitation algorithm*

- *feel* for carotid and femoral pulses if peripheral radial pulses are not present. Assess for rate, quality (weak/thready/strong), regularity and equality. Examine for swelling, distension or painful areas that may indicate internal bleeding or ischaemia. Feel for changes in skin temperature and assess capillary refill.

> **Practice point**
> Listen to the heart: normal heart sounds or gallop rhythm? Is there a new murmur?

> **Practice point**
> Most unwell surgical patients will benefit from oxygen and fluid therapy while you are performing your assessment.

Full patient assessment

CHART REVIEW

The notes and charts contain a lot of data. Again, a systematic approach minimises the chance of missing important facts. Sometimes, it can be useful to complete your note and chart review before speaking in detail to the ward nurses and doctors. This gives a fresh opinion and provides you with a factual base for discussing the patient. The notes will provide basic clinical information on premorbid status, comorbidity and any procedures performed. On the charts, look at both the absolute values and the trends. Absolute values are notoriously unreliable and more useful information can be obtained by looking at trends over the preceding few hours. The charts should indicate the progress of the patient; parameters that may be measured include:

- respiratory rate, oxygen FiO_2 and saturation;
- heart rate and rhythm;
- blood pressure: systolic/diastolic;
- CVP (if being measured);
- temperature;
- urinary output;
- intravenous lines: position and condition;
- fluid therapy: prescribed versus given; and
- drainage of all types.

Review the drug chart for drugs causing CVS change (given/omitted).

Respiratory rate

- The most sensitive marker of the 'ill' patient and often the first parameter to change as the patient deteriorates.
- Accurate observation and recording are essential.
- Rates below 11/min may be due to opiate/sedative overdose or other causes of central nervous system depression, including low cardiac output.
- A high respiratory rate is an early sign of many kinds of shock, as well as respiratory disease or cardiac failure.

Heart rate and rhythm

- There is enormous individual variation with age and disease.
- Interpret absolute values of pulse rate along with coexisting medical conditions or drug treatment: beware the patient on beta-blockers or who has a pacemaker. In both cases, the normal cardiac response to hypovolaemia or pyrexia will be blocked.
- Tachycardia can be an early sign of shock.
- Acute dysrhythmia is an important sign of myocardial failure or ischaemia.

Blood pressure

- Changes in both systolic and diastolic blood pressure are often late signs but when present should flag up the severity of the underlying problem.
- Think perfusion rather than pressure: a high or normal blood pressure with poor perfusion is of no help to the patient.
- Remember that for the elderly patient who usually runs at 180/100 mmHg, a pressure of 110/70 mmHg represents significant hypotension and may be inadequate.

> **Practice point**
> Clinical signs may be unreliable in that normal values do not exclude significant abnormality, *but* abnormal values should be acted upon!

Jugular venous pressure/central venous pressure

- Jugular venous distension measured with the patient at 45 degrees in the sitting position will give a clinical indication of the CVP.
- Collapsed neck veins with the patient at 45 degrees indicates low jugular venous pressure (JVP).

- JVP not visible with the patient flat is always abnormal.
- Trends in CVP measurement, particularly the response to a fluid bolus, are much more useful than absolute values.
- Consider formal CVP monitoring early in ill patients when management of fluids is becoming problematic.

ABNORMALITIES OF CVP

A low CVP:

- may be due to inadequate fluid therapy;
- may be an indication of continued bleeding;
- may be due to vasodilation in response to sepsis;
- must be corrected in the face of hypotension;
- may be associated with a low cardiac output;
- may be explained by vasodilation due to epidural analgesia – exclude other causes.

A high CVP may be:

- temporary following a rapid fluid bolus;
- a result of fluid overload;
- due to right ventricular failure as a result of myocardial infarction or pulmonary embolism;
- due to congestive cardiac failure (CCF);
- due to pulmonary hypertension (which may be long-standing);
- caused by pericardial effusion with tamponade.

If in any doubt as to the cause or treatment required, seek expert help.

Temperature

- May be high (>38°C) or low (<36°C) in sepsis or systemic inflammatory response syndrome (SIRS) but may be normal even in the presence of severe intra-abdominal sepsis in the immunocompromised, the elderly and patients on steroids.
- Core/peripheral (rectal/axillary) temperature difference of more than 2°C suggests poor peripheral perfusion.
- Low-grade pyrexia occurs after myocardial infarction, in bacterial endocarditis (irregular, mild, accompanied by a cardiac murmur and anaemia) and with diurnal variation in a warm environment (highest in the early evening).

Urinary output

- Probably the best surrogate marker of cardiac output and tissue perfusion that is readily available on the ward.

- The hypoxic or underperfused kidney does not perform well and is an excellent marker of early cardiovascular problems.
- Look for a steady decline to indicate a problem rather than sudden complete anuria, which suggests a blocked catheter.

Intravenous lines

- Those inserted during emergency resuscitation are more likely to be infected. Even peripheral lines are a potential source of sepsis.
- Placement is difficult in shocked patients, and often the existing line is too small to deliver an adequate rate of fluid.
- Tissued lines cause morbidity both from the local effect of extravasated fluids and drugs and systemically as a result of the failure of the fluid and drugs to reach the circulation.

Tubes and drains

- These may or may not be patent.
- Sudden occlusion of chest drains may lead to tension pneumothorax.
- Pericardial drains occluding after cardiac surgery may cause cardiac tamponade.
- Occluded abdominal drains may allow bleeding to remain hidden for some time before diagnosis.
- Drainage volumes and nasogastric aspirate are an essential part of fluid balance calculations.

Drug chart review

- This may reveal that regular cardiac drugs have been missed while the patient was 'nil by mouth'.
- Alternatively, drugs may have been administered that have produced adverse cardiovascular effects as a result of overdosage, accumulation or interaction with other systems, *eg* steroids preventing pyrexia in sepsis or masking abdominal signs.

Fluid balance

- Determine type and quantity of fluids given and the fluid balance for the current 24 hours and the preceding days.
- Has the fluid been given as prescribed (often inadequate, slow or curtailed)?
- It is much more frequent for unwell surgical patients to be hypovolaemic, but colloids are occasionally given in large amounts during initial resuscitation and can overload patients with cardiac disease.

- Pulmonary oedema may be iatrogenic, particularly in the elderly patient, and may result from 'fluid creep', *ie* several consecutive days with a positive fluid balance.
- Remember that all patients are different and do not respond identically to apparently similar fluid regimens: we treat more 'typical' surgical patients than examples of '*Homo physiologicus*' (see Table 4.1). Fluid requirements can be determined only by regular review and reassessment.

HISTORY

Taking a careful and detailed history from the patient and from the notes will help to identify cardiac problems. Remember that nursing colleagues and relatives can be useful additional sources of information. Specific points worth remembering include:

- speed of onset and duration of any symptoms;
- pain: its nature, severity, site and radiations;
- presence of dyspnoea; and
- functional exercise tolerance.

CASE NOTES

From the notes, determine:

- *admission:* reason(s) for;
- *operative procedure(s)*, and if so what;
- *anaesthetic(s):* method and any untoward problems;
- *past history* of myocardial infarction (MI), CCF, cardiac surgery, exercise tolerance, angina, syncope, nocturnal dyspnoea, hypertension, rheumatic fever; and
- *medication:* present and past.

EXAMINATION

Utilise all the available clinical information and *think perfusion*.

Look

- *Overview:* is the patient alert? confused? restless? moribund? (ABCs!).
- *Colour:* presence of peripheral or central cyanosis, anaemia.
- *Peripheries:* assess for peripheral perfusion and presence of oedema.
- *Neck veins.*

Listen

Breath sounds:

- Assess for the presence of basal crepitations, indicative of left-sided failure.
- In early left-sided failure, bronchial wheeze (cardiac asthma) may be present, due to small airway narrowing as a result of pulmonary oedema.

Heart sounds:

- Assess for the presence of added sounds or murmurs (?new).
- Time the murmur with the carotid pulse: remember a diastolic murmur is never 'physiological'.

Feel

- *Skin:* may feel clammy with poor capillary filling in cardiogenic shock.
- *Liver:* assess for presence of hepatomegaly or ascites, which may be an indication of congestive heart failure. Heart failure can cause abdominal pain from acute distension of the liver capsule.

AVAILABLE RESULTS

Include the available results and previous investigations in your assessment. Remember that ward care is different to HDU/ICU care and it is unlikely

Table 4.1 *Differences between* Homo physiologicus *(physiology textbook man) and* Homo octogenarius chirurgiae *(typical surgical patient)*

Homo physiologicus	*Homo octogenarius chirurgiae*
70 kg, 180 cm tall	35–110 kg, related inversely to height
Two kidneys	One kidney (slightly damaged)
Resting cardiac output 5 l/min: increases significantly when needed	Cardiac output indeterminable: MI three years ago, on thiazides since; occasionally walks dog
Healthy lungs	Smoked 20/day for 20 years
No comorbidity	Three days of vomiting; now has peritonitis

Table 4.2 *Indicators of low cardiac output*

Cool, clammy skin with poor capillary flushing
Rapid, low-volume pulse
Peripheral cyanosis
Low peripheral temperature or core/peripheral temperature
 gradient >2°C
Oliguria or anuria
Confusion
Metabolic acidaemia

that the complete range of cardiovascular tests will have been performed. Be realistic, look at what is available, and use the findings of your clinical examination, note and chart review to determine whether any further specific tests are required. Demanding unnecessary tests is time-consuming and costly and inflicts further discomfort.

As a minimum to aid your assessment, look at the most recent haemoglobin, white cell count, platelet count and electrolytes and urea, and compare them with those taken when the patient was well. If no contemporary results are available since deterioration, these will need to be ordered. Additional tests will be necessary if you suspect particular problems, *eg* cardiac enzymes for MI.

Blood results

Haemoglobin:

- Anaemia may precipitate failure in the cardiac patient and caution will be required during transfusion. Diuretic cover may be needed (but not always – consider cardiac function and volume state).
- Oxygen transport to the tissues is optimal at a haemoglobin value around 10 g/dl; at higher values, viscosity reduces microcirculatory flow.

A *leukocytosis* may be present following MI.

Hypokalaemia:

- Hypokalaemia can impair myocardial function, particularly in the patient on digoxin.
- ECG changes may occur (U waves), but there is poor correlation between the changes and magnitude of the potassium depletion.
- A decrease in serum potassium of 1 mmol/l reflects a total body deficit of 200–300 mmol/l.
- Give KCl at a rate of no more than 20 mmol/l/h, with ECG monitoring and regular monitoring of plasma potassium concentration.

Hyperkalaemia:

- Levels of 7 mmol/l and above will produce ECG changes (widespread peaked T waves).
- Treatment (see Table 4.3) must be *immediate* if levels of this magnitude are found, as hyperkalaemia can lead to dysrhythmias and death.

Table 4.3 *Temporary treatments for hyperkalaemia*

Calcium gluconate or chloride 1 g i.v. over 10–15 minutes
Correct any acidosis by giving NaHCO₃ – watch for
 hypernatraemia
Glucose 50% – 50 ml containing insulin 10 units given by
 syringe pump over 30–60 minutes
Intravenous salbutamol infusion can be used, but it may cause
 a tachycardia
ECG monitoring is mandatory for all of the above

Hypernatraemia and calcium disturbances: sodium acts as a myocardial depressant, and low or high levels of calcium cause ECG changes.

Hypomagnesaemia is common and is associated with dysrhythmias (see later).

Cardiac enzymes and troponin (see below) should be checked serially to exclude MI. *Thyroid function tests* will be required occasionally.

Chest X-ray

The chest X-ray can help differentiate respiratory conditions from cardiovascular conditions and aids in the positive identification of heart failure in particular. A system for looking at X-rays is outlined in Chapter 3.

The electrocardiograph

As with other investigations, the ECG should never be looked at in isolation; it should be interpreted in light of the clinical findings. It may show nothing significant, even in the failing heart, but it is important to be able to recognise common patterns. As most bedside monitors do not show a trace adequate for accurate diagnosis, a formal 12-lead ECG must be obtained for analysis. Instruction and practice in the interpretation of ECGs and the management of common dysrhythmias in surgical patients will be given during the practical course.

INTERPRETING THE ECG

Objectives

- To learn a system for examining ECGs.
- To be aware of the common important abnormalities in critically ill surgical patients.
- To know the initial treatment of common cardiac dysrhythmias.

Always work to a routine when looking at an ECG (see Table 4.4). Check the patient's name, date and time, and compare with old ECGs.

Rotation of the heart and morphology of the precordial QRS complexes

See Fig. 4.2. The size of the R wave in V1 increases progressively towards V6 because the underlying myocardium becomes progressively thicker over the left ventricle. Note that depolarisation occurs from endocardium to epicardium and this reflects myocardial thickness. Occasionally, the R wave in V6 may be smaller than in V5 and that in V5 is smaller than in V4; this is because the electrodes in these leads are further away from the myocardium than in V1–V3 in these cases.

The size of the S wave (first negative deflection after the R wave) tends to decrease towards V6.

The direction of the first part of the QRS complex is upwards in V1–V3 (an R wave), but this becomes a negative deflection as it progresses to V6 (Q wave). This is not pathological and is due to rotation of the heart about a near-vertical axis (left hip to right shoulder), thus producing a variation in the relative positions of the two ventricles. This rotation causing the variations in QRS complexes is not clinically significant and is dependent on the individual.

Since the height of the R wave and the depth of the S wave are influenced by the thickness of the underlying myocardium, these deflections will be abnormally large in conditions producing hypertrophy, *eg* left ventricular hypertrophy secondary to hypertension or aortic valve disease. However, in the thin patient, the R wave may be 'abnormally' high over V4–V6.

Electrical axis of the heart

The spread of depolarisation across the myocardium produces 'vector loops' of electrical activity. When the depolarisation wave moves towards an electrode, an upward or positive deflection will be recorded. Conversely, moving away from an electrode will produce a downward or negative deflection. The angle at which this electrical wave moves in relationship to a particular electrode will determine the degree of upward or downward deflection recorded by it. Each lead of the ECG 'looks' at the heart from a different aspect, or 'angle'. These angles can be displayed using the Hexaxial Reference System.

Figure 4.3 shows the angle of the heart that each bipolar lead sees. By comparing the relative heights of the R wave and the depth of the S wave, the electrical axis, or sum of the depolarisation vectors, can be determined. Basically, the more the electrical axis points towards an electrode, the greater the deflection produced by that electrode; see leads II and F in Fig. 4.3a and leads L and I in Fig. 4.3b.

This description is simplified and is intended only to give you an outline of the subject.

What is the electrical axis in the example shown in Fig. 4.4?

'Normal' ranges in ECG interpretation

The 'normal' ranges in ECG interpretation are shown in Table 4.5 and Figs 4.5 and 4.6.

Table 4.4 *Routine for looking at an ECG*

Axis	Use deflection in bipolar leads	
Rhythm	Use the R wave (lead II)	?Regular
Rate	Use the R wave	?Normal
P wave	Presence and morphology	?Sinus rhythm
PR interval	Short	Pre-excitation, *eg* WPW
	Long	*eg* heart block
QRS complex	Height, width, presence of Q waves	?MI, ?BBB
ST segment	Depressed or elevated	?MI, ?ischaemia, ?digitalis toxicity
T wave	Height, shape	?Ischaemia, ?biochemical abnormalities
U wave	Presence	?Hypokalaemia

BBB, bundle branch block; WPW, Wolff–Parkinson–White syndrome

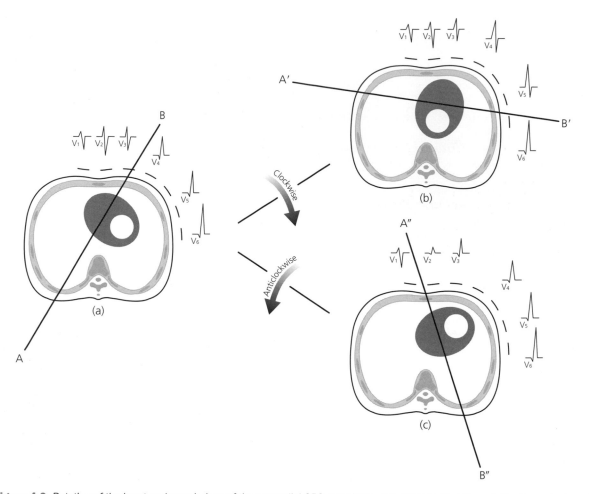

Figure 4.2 *Rotation of the heart and morphology of the precordial QRS complexes. The cross-section through the thorax is viewed from below. (a) Intermediate position. (b) Clockwise rotation. (c) Anticlockwise rotation*

Decide, plan and treat

The clinical assessment and investigations described above should lead to a diagnosis that explains the patient's deterioration. The next task is to reach a decision based on the findings and, if need be, to arrange any necessary investigations or specialist opinions. Make a management plan to treat the problem and prevent recurrence. Conditions that do not resolve rapidly with relatively simple measures will require expert help and a higher level of care. After any intervention, you will need to **reassess** and modify the management plan.

Remember that the CVS has considerable reserve: by the time dysfunction is evident, the problems are marked. Do not leave a patient with an obviously compromised CVS – they won't be there when you get back!

SPECIFIC MANAGEMENT PROBLEMS

Diagnosis and management of hypotension

Although hypotension is the commonest cardiovascular problem seen in surgical critical care patients, it has been discussed in Chapter 2 and will be explored further in Chapter 5.

Diagnosis and management of tachyarrhythmias

Being called to evaluate a surgical patient with a tachycardia is common (see Table 4.6). Management initially follows the system of assessment. A patient with unstable vital signs needs prompt diagnosis and treatment. At the other end of the spectrum,

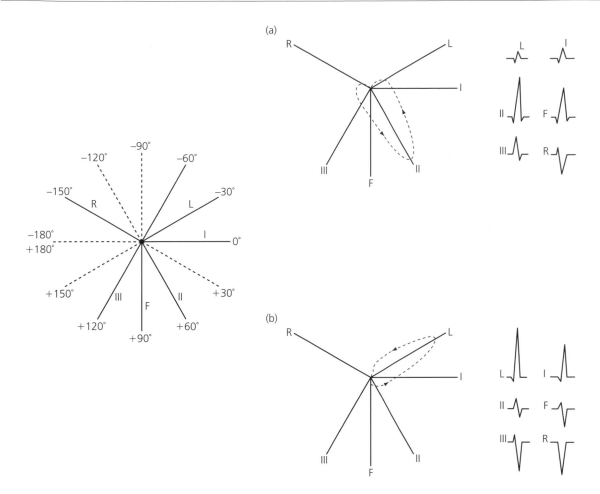

Figure 4.3 *Electrical axis of the heart*

longstanding, asymptomatic atrial fibrillation (AF) is common in the elderly and might simply need the correction of fluid balance or the reinstitution of routine digoxin treatment. Usually, some action will be required. If any doubt exists, ask for senior help.

The type of tachycardia will be evident only from the ECG.

TREATMENT

A systematic approach to the problem should be adopted. Start with the ABCs: correct hypoxia, hypovolaemia and electrolyte disturbances.

Carotid sinus massage (CSM) and Valsalva manoeuvres may correct a supraventricular tachycardia, but this is unlikely to be permanent.

Drugs:
- Care must be taken with all drugs, particularly in patients with poor ventricular function or hypotension.

- Only use a drug if you are familiar with both its actions and its side effects.
- *If there is any doubt about a drug, then it should not be given*, and help must be sought.
- Remember that in the longer term, if atrial fibrillation or flutter persists, then anticoagulation will be necessary in order to prevent emboli.

DC cardioversion:
- DC conversion should be considered early when there is a very rapid rate or evidence of compromise.
- The patient must be anaesthetised.
- DC conversion is less effective in cases of longstanding atrial arrhythmias.
- Appropriate help must be sought at an early stage.

The use of *pacing and surgical ablation* is beyond the scope of this manual. These techniques should be used as a last resort under the guidance of a cardiologist.

Table 4.5 'Normal' ECG ranges

At 25 mm/s	Large square $= 0.2$ s
	Small square $= 0.04$ s
QRS width	Normal: < 0.12 s
	Wide: 0.12 s
Tachycardia	Ventricular rate > 100 bpm
Bradycardia	Ventricular rate < 60 bpm
Electrical axis	$+90$ to -30
	Vertical: $+60$ to $+90$ (tall individuals)
	Intermediate: $+30$ to $+60$
	Horizontal: $+30$ to -30 (stocky, squat individuals)
	Axis shifts towards the left in the elderly
T wave	Normally upright, except in aVR; inversion can also occur in III, V1 and V2
P wave	Normally upright
	Inversion can occur in retrograde P waves in atrioventricular (AV) nodal rhythm
	Tall, peaked waves in pulmonary hypertension ('pulmonary P')
	Biphasic in mitral valve disease ('mitral P')
PR interval	Measured from the start of the P wave to the first deflection of the QRS complex, whether it is upright to inverted
	Range: 0.12–0.2 s
QT interval	Variable, depends on rate
Q wave	First downward (negative) deflection after the P wave
	Normal in leads III and aVR and sometimes in leads V4, V5 and V6
	Width no more than 0.04 s duration
	Depth no more than one-quarter the height of the following R wave
U wave	Normal when T wave is normal, but in hypokalaemia it may become more prominent as the T wave flattens

ALGORITHM OF MANAGEMENT

- Check and correct ABCs. Cardiopulmonary resuscitation (CPR) or immediate anaesthetic and cardiology support may be necessary. It is better to summon help *before* arrest occurs. Be guided by experienced nursing staff.
- Use 12-lead ECG to allow accurate diagnosis and exclude MI.

Table 4.6 Causes of tachycardia

Trauma	Hypovolaemia, anaemia, contused myocardium
Inflammatory	Pyrexia, pericarditis
Metabolic	Acidosis
Haematological	Anaemia
Circulatory	Shock from any cause, arrhythmias, pulmonary embolism, MI
Endocrine	Thyrotoxicosis
Drugs	Aminophylline, digitalis toxicity, beta agonists
Anxiety and pain	

- Rule out/correct hypovolaemia, hypoxia, hypokalaemia and hypomagnesaemia.
- Check that routine medications have been given.

Adenosine

If the diagnosis is not clear after clinical and ECG interpretation, then the administration of adenosine (0.05–0.25 mg/kg) can be revealing. Adenosine has a powerful blocking effect on the atrioventricular (AV) node, thus slowing the ventricular rate if the dysrhythmia is atrial in origin. It acts for only 15–20 seconds and is relatively safe in experi-

Table 4.7 Causes of arrhythmia

Ischaemic heart disease
Oxygen, fluid and electrolyte disturbances
Drugs
Rheumatic heart disease
Cardiomyopathy
Thyrotoxicosis

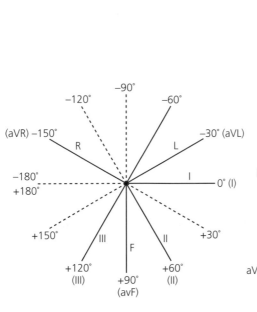

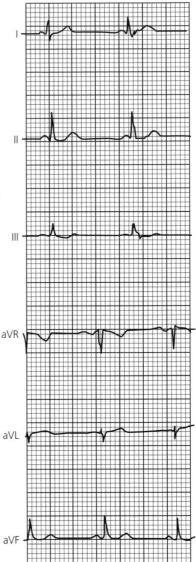

Figure 4.4 *An electrical axis*

enced hands. Its use should be avoided in asthmatic patients and in the presence of dipyridamole, as dipyridamole greatly prolongs the action of adenosine.

Case history 4.1

A 73-year-old man, a known hypertensive who usually takes amlodipine, underwent anterior resection for carcinoma of the rectum this morning. You review him at 8pm on the evening of surgery and find him to be in atrial fibrillation, with a rate of 90 bpm. This developed about 30 minutes previously.

On your immediate assessment, you find that the patient appears quite well; he tells you that he feels comfortable (he has an epidural infusion in progress). His respiratory rate is 18/min, and his oxygen saturation is reading 97% with facemask oxygen at 40%. You examine him and find that his peripheries are well perfused. His blood pressure is unchanged from preoperatively at 150/80 mmHg. Your initial assessment reveals no other findings.

You review his charts and notes and find that his urine output has been only 40 ml over the last two hours. His CVP has been decreasing gradually since return from theatre and is now reading 2 mmHg. He was prescribed two units of blood to run over three

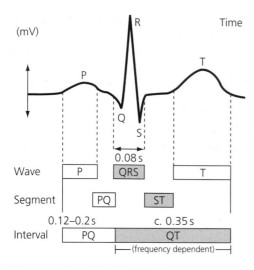

Figure 4.5 *Normal annotated PQRST*

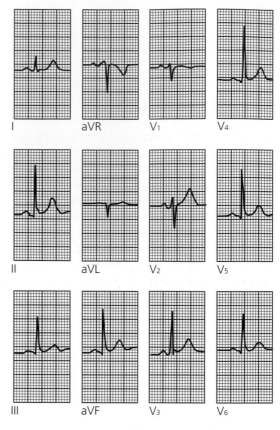

Figure 4.6 *Normal ECG trace*

hours each, followed by 1000 ml saline eight-hourly by the anaesthetist. The first litre of saline has just been started.

You ask the nurse to give the patient the litre of saline over one hour, and check a full blood count and his urea and electrolytes. His haemoglobin is satisfactory at 110 g/l. His serum potassium is 3.2 mmol/l. All other electrolytes, including magnesium, are within normal limits. You prescribe 20 mmol of potassium to be given in 100 ml saline over the next hour and arrange with the sister in charge of the HDU to review him in an hour. When you review him, he is in sinus rhythm, with a rate of 75 bpm, his CVP has risen to 6 mmHg and he has passed 30 ml of urine over the past 30 minutes. You change the fluid prescription to 1,000 ml saline with 20 mmol KCl per litre six-hourly, and you arrange to review the patient again later that evening.

Learning points

- Use the CCrISP system of assessment to review all patients.
- Regular review of patients at risk will lead to early detection of potential problems.
- Correction of hypovolaemia, hypoxia and electrolyte disturbances is simple but often very effective.

VENTRICULAR TACHYCARDIAS

These are potentially malignant rhythms that require *prompt specialist referral*. Cardioversion is often required. Amiodarone (5 mg/kg over 20 min) may be useful.

VENTRICULAR ECTOPICS

Ventricular ectopics (VEs) may be unifocal (each ectopic having the same shape) or multifocal (each ectopic having a different shape). The pulse will be irregular. An ECG is the only certain way to distinguish this from other causes of irregular pulse (see Table 4.8). The danger lies in the fact that an ectopic arising on the apex of a T wave will produce ventricular fibrillation. Clearly, the more ectopics there are,

Table 4.8 *Differentiating supraventricular tachycardia (SVT) and ventricular tachycardia (VT): some pointers*

SVT	VT
QRS narrow complex	Often broad complex
Often no P waves	P waves, dissociated rhythm
Usually regular	May be irregular
QRS right way up	QRS inverted
May respond to carotid sinus massage (CSM)	No response to CSM
Slowed with adenosine	No response to adenosine

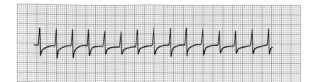

Figure 4.7 *Supraventricular tachycardia*

the greater is the probability of this happening. Treatment should be considered if the ratio of VE to normal QRS is greater than 1 : 6 or if multifocal. Lidocaine (lignocaine) is the treatment of choice.

Clinical association: VEs can occur in healthy people without evidence of any disease. The incidence is higher in older individuals. VEs also occur after MI, with electrolyte disturbance, *eg* hypokalaemia and hypomagnesaemia, in valvular heart disease, with cardiomyopathies, with hypoxia and in digitalis toxicity.

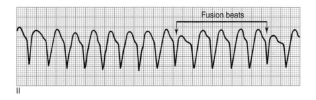

Figure 4.8 *Ventricular tachycardia*

Common types of atrial tachycardia

SINUS TACHYCARDIA

- Regular up to 160/min or so in young patients.
- Lesser maximum rate in older patients.
- Normal P and morphology.
- Gradual onset.
- Treat cause: hypovolaemia, anaemia, pulmonary embolism, sepsis, etc.

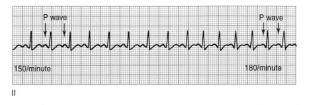

Figure 4.9 *Sinus tachycardia*

PAROXYSMAL SUPRAVENTRICULAR TACHYCARDIA

- Any tachycardia originating in the AV node, atria or sinoatrial (SA) node.

- P waves can be of abnormal shape and may or may not be seen.
- QRS width usually normal (may be wide if associated bundle branch block).
- May be associated with ST depression, suggesting ischaemia.
- Regular 150–250/min.
- Abolished/slowed by CSM and adenosine.
- *Treatment:* verapamil, digoxin, beta-blockade (avoid in heart failure or with verapamil).

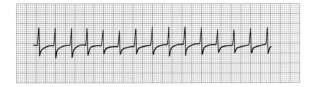

Figure 4.10 *Paroxysmal SVT*

ATRIAL FIBRILLATION

- Irregularly irregular, variable ventricular rate, often 100–180/min.
- Very common postoperatively in surgical patients.
- Associated with hypovolaemia, hypoxia and electrolyte disorders.
- Also associated with cardiopulmonary disease (*eg* ischaemic or rheumatic heart disease).
- No P waves, normal QRS.

The management of atrial fibrillation (AF) depends on its cause and its effects.

Many new cases occur after surgery and are caused by hypovolaemia, hypoxia or electrolyte imbalance, particularly hypokalaemia and hypomagnesaemia. These episodes can be treated rapidly by correcting the causal factors alone, and such problems should always be corrected rapidly in all cases. Look for and treat any underlying problems that would cause these factors to recur.

When new AF causes **serious adverse signs** (particularly hypotension, shock, chest pain, heart

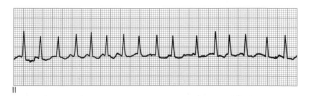

Figure 4.11 *Atrial fibrillation*

failure, decreased conscious level or marked tachy-cardia >140/min), urgent treatment is needed, with DC cardioversion or with intravenous amiodarone. Expert help is needed directly.

New AF that does not cause serious adverse signs and that does not respond to the correction of general factors is most commonly treated with digoxin or amiodarone. However, if problems persist or recur or are beyond your competence, then get expert help.

Longstanding AF can worsen after surgery if the usual drugs have been omitted. In such cases, you are unlikely to convert the patient back to sinus rhythm, and rate control with digoxin or amiodarone is usually needed. Ultimately, you may have to consider anticoagulation.

- Correct general causes as above, particularly hypoxia, hypovolaemia and hypomagnesaemia.
- DC cardioversion: consider when the patient is acutely decompensated or following recent onset (more responsive).
- Digoxin 0.25–0.5 mg if reversal is not urgent.
- Amiodarone 5 mg/kg over 20 minutes (care with digoxin!).

ATRIAL FLUTTER

- Regular flutter P waves 300/min.
- Regular normal QRS, variable AV block.
- Usually associated with cardiac disease.
- May respond to CSM; adenosine may reveal flutter waves.
- Atrial flutter and fibrillation may be present in the same patient.
- *Treatment:* cardioversion, digoxin, verapamil (care with digoxin!).

Remember, always investigate the cause!

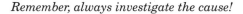
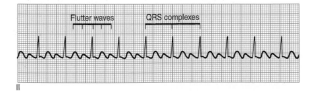

Figure 4.12 *Atrial flutter with 3 : 1 AV block*

Left ventricular hypertrophy

A hypertrophied left ventricle has a greater influence on the electrical axis of the heart and causes

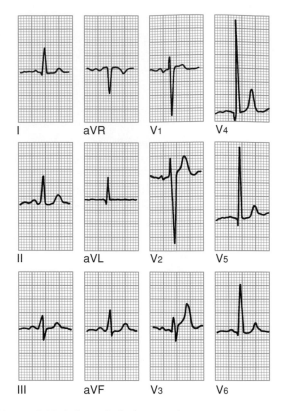

Figure 4.13 *Left ventricular hypertrophy*

left axis deviation. This gives the picture of tall R waves in leads I and aVL and S waves in leads III and aVF. Most noticeably, the increase in the left ventricular muscle mass also produces tall R waves in leads over the left ventricle (V4–V6) and deep S waves in leads over the right ventricle (V1–V3).

Clinical associations: conditions causing an increase in afterload or work on the left ventricle, *eg* aortic valve disease, systemic hypertension.

Right ventricular hypertrophy

When the electrical activity of the hypertrophied right ventricle predominates over the left, there is right axis deviation (leads I, II, III) with a tall R wave in V1 and a deep S wave in V6. A tall 'pulmonary P' wave suggests right atrial hypertrophy.

Clinical associations: conditions causing increased right ventricular afterload, *eg* pulmonary hypertension, cor pulmonale, pulmonary stenosis.

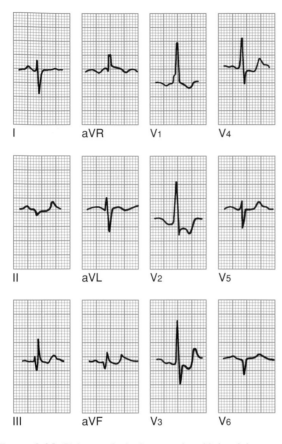

Figure 4.14 *Right ventricular hypertrophy with 'strain'*

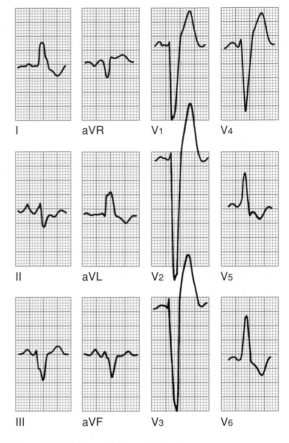

Figure 4.15 *Left bundle branch block*

Left bundle branch block

Electrical activity in the left ventricle is delayed because conduction to it must take place via the right ventricle. The resultant delay in left ventricular depolarisation produces the M-shaped QRS wave, typically in leads V5, V6, I and aVL, and a W-shaped QRS in some of the reciprocal leads, typically leads III and aVF (Fig. 4.15).

Right bundle branch block

Conversely, in right bundle branch block, right ventricular depolarisation occurs via the left ventricle. In right bundle branch block, the M-shaped QRS is typically in leads V1, V2 and V3. Right bundle branch block with left axis deviation suggests bifascicular block. This condition will often need pacing: seek help early!

Clinical associations: coronary artery disease, valvular heart disease, ventricular hypertrophy and fibrosis, cardiomyopathies.

Bradyarrhythmias

Slow heart rates are problematic if they are associated with hypoperfusion or hypotension. They are common in the elderly (Table 4.9). The patient likely to get troublesome heart block (*eg* those with bifascicular block) should be detected preoperatively and considered for elective pacing.

In the patient with symptomatic bradycardia, atropine (0.6–1.2 mg) may help, but pacing may be needed. Isoprenaline infusion may be used under the guidance of an intensivist or cardiologist. Discuss with your medical or ICU colleagues sooner rather than later!

Myocardial infarction

Ischaemic heart disease is very common, particularly in the elderly and in patients with peripheral or cerebrovascular disease or diabetes mellitus. Perioperative MI has a higher mortality than that

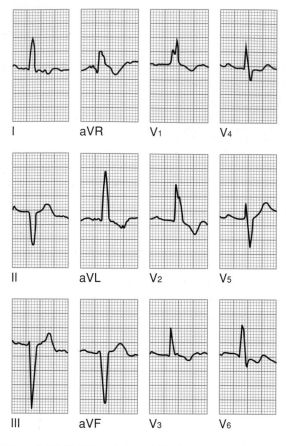

I	aVR	V1	V4
II	aVL	V2	V5
III	aVF	V3	V6

Figure 4.16 *Right bundle branch block*

occurring remote from operation. A recent MI (within six months) should preclude elective surgery, since the incidence of perioperative MI is increased within this period. All cardiac drugs should be continued up to and including the day of operation and recommended at the earliest opportunity postoperatively. Perioperative MI often is silent

Table 4.9 *Conditions associated with bradycardia*

Autonomic
    Pain, especially visceral (may also be associated with tachycardia)
    Raised intracranial pressure
    Drugs: beta-blockers
Non-autonomic
    MI (particularly inferior MI)
    Gram-negative sepsis
    Hypoxia
    Drugs: digitalis toxicity
    Hypothyroidism
    Hypothermia

or presents with shortness of breath, hypotension, evidence of decreased organ function (including confusion) secondary to cardiogenic shock, acute dysrhythmias, sudden pulmonary oedema or cardiac arrest. It enters the differential diagnosis of acute upper abdominal pain. A high index of suspicion is required, particularly in high-risk groups.

The ECG may show typical changes of anterior, anterolateral or inferior MI with ST segment elevation of more than 1 mm in the relevant leads overlying the infarct (primary changes), and inversion in the leads opposite to it (reciprocal changes). T waves flatten and invert within hours to days of MI, and Q waves develop over one to two days (see Table 4.10). Changes may be masked by a preexisting left bundle branch block, and new bundle branch block should make you suspicious. *The ECG may be normal after an MI, particularly for the first hour or so.* A normal ECG therefore does not exclude MI.

Table 4.10 *Time of ECG changes after MI*

Change	Onset/duration
Peaked T waves	Seconds
ST changes (usually elevation)	Hours
Q waves	Hours/days
T-wave inversion	Hours/days

Practice point

Recognition of patterns of ECG changes in MI:

- Anterior infarct: primary changes V1, V2, V3, V4.
- Inferior infarct: primary changes II, III, aVF.
- Posterior infarct: isolated ST depression V1, V2.

Treatment: oxygen, analgesia, refer and transfer to high care area.

Early treatment influences the outcome significantly. If you suspect the presence of an MI, then seek the advice of a physician urgently.

In the meantime:

- Check and correct the ABCs.
- Make your patient comfortable with a suitable opiate analgesic. Morphine (or diamorphine) is best, titrated to response intravenously (1 to 2-mg

boluses every two minutes). Cyclizine (50 mg) or metoclopramide (10 mg) intravenously can be used to prevent or treat nausea.

- Give high-flow oxygen to reduce hypoxia (monitor SaO_2).
- Give glyceryl trinitrate (sublingual or spray) to reduce coronary artery spasm. Nitrates also have a synergistic effect with thrombolysis.
- Arrange appropriate investigations:
  - ECG (serial ECGs are required)
  - blood tests to exclude anaemia and electrolyte disturbances, for cardiac enzymes and troponin levels (if available locally).

ECG changes of MI are localised to ischaemic or infarcted areas, whereas generalised changes are seen in, for example, hyperkalaemia (peaked T waves) or pericarditis (ST elevation).

ANTERIOR MYOCARDIAL INFARCTION

Raised ST segments in V1–V4.

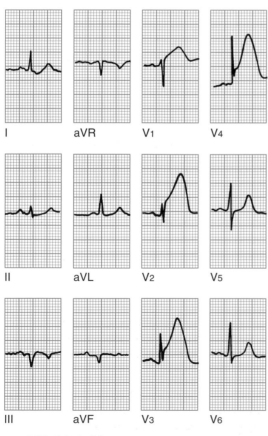

Figure 4.17 *Anterior MI*

INFERIOR MYOCARDIAL INFARCTION

Raised ST segments and Q waves can be seen in leads II, III and aVF (with reciprocal ST depression in leads I, aVL and V2–V4). Non-pathological Q waves may be present in leads II and III. Compare this with anterior MI.

Further treatment may involve the use of:

- *Aspirin:* 150–300 mg.
- *Fibrinolytics:* streptokinase or alteplase (rTPA) can be used, particularly if there is persistent chest pain and gross ECG changes. Contraindications to fibrinolytics include:
  - immediate postoperative period (<2 weeks)
  - previous streptokinase treatment (further streptokinase contraindicated; use rTPA)
  - active peptic ulcer
  - previous haemorrhagic stroke
  - recent head injury, however minor
  - prolonged traumatic cardiopulmonary resuscitation.
- *Beta-blockers:* providing there is no evidence of cardiac failure, bradycardia or hypotension, beta-

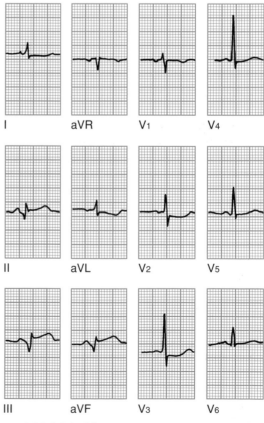

Figure 4.18 *Inferior MI*

blockers such as atenolol (up to 15 mg in 5-mg boluses) have been shown to improve survival by reducing the incidence of cardiac rupture. Their use may also help in cases of ventricular tachycardia, which is associated with large infarcts and an increased risk of ventricular fibrillation.

- *Angioplasty and coronary stenting:* alternatives available in specialist centres. Urgent referral is needed, because the success of these treatments can be time-critical. Your hospital will have a protocol for the management of acute coronary syndromes, and you should discuss possible cases at an early stage.

Acute coronary syndromes

'Acute coronary syndrome' is an increasingly used all-encompassing term that refers to a variety of myocardial conditions, including acute MI (both Q-wave and non-Q-wave) and unstable angina. The full range of conditions is listed in Table 4.11.

Table 4.11 *Acute coronary syndromes*

Acute MI
transmural MI
Q-wave MI
STEMI
Non-Q-wave MI
subendocardial infarction
non-STEMI
Unstable angina

STEMI, ST elevation myocardial infarction

In most of these patients, the development of an acute coronary syndrome is due to rupture or erosion of an atherosclerotic plaque within the walls of a coronary artery, leading to thrombus formation. This is followed by platelet aggregation and vasoconstriction of the associated vessels. Less commonly, an acute coronary syndrome is the result of emboli or coronary spasm. It is often impossible to distinguish between the different causes clinically.

TREATMENT STRATEGIES

As the principal problem in most patients is the disruption of coronary blood flow due to the formation of thrombus within the coronary vessel, therapeutic intervention is directed towards clot removal and prevention of its re-accumulation and the resulting restoration of coronary blood flow. In the case of Q-wave MI, it is now well established that aspirin and fibrinolytic therapy leading to immediate revascularisation are the first-line therapies. In non-Q-wave infarction, fibrinolytic treatment is not used, but antiplatelet agents such as aspirin and, more recently, the glycoprotein IIb/IIIa antagonists have been shown to confer some benefit.

Congestive cardiac failure

CCF is common in surgical critical care. It varies in severity from mild dyspnoea that is treated easily to cardiogenic shock. Demands on the heart are increased by surgical illness, and this may unmask or worsen cardiac failure.

Cardiac function depends on preload, intrinsic myocardial function and afterload. This concept can be simplified in the following way: if the heart is thought of as a simple pump, the preload is analogous to the priming of the pump; it will work well only if it has something (but not too much) to pump. Ensuring adequate cardiac filling is essential. Any condition that disturbs pump filling will affect preload and therefore cardiac function (see Table 4.12, point a).

Table 4.12 *Causes of cardiac failure in surgical critical care*

(a) Conditions affecting preload
Hypovolaemia (bleeding, inadequate volume replacement, etc)
Fluid overload
Pneumothorax/cardiac tamponade (see also points b and c below)
(b) Conditions affecting intrinsic myocardial function
Ischaemia
Infarction
Dysrhythmias
Chronic heart failure + operative stress
Hypocalcaemia and other electrolyte disturbances
Myocardial depressant factors, eg in sepsis
Pneumothorax/cardiac tamponade (see also points a and c)
(c) Conditions affecting afterload
Aortic/pulmonary valvular stenosis
Pulmonary embolism
Pneumothorax/cardiac tamponade (see also points a and b above)
Aortic dissection

Intrinsic myocardial function is analogous to the function of the pump itself; if the pump fails in any way, it will not be able to cope with the demands made on it. Any condition that directly affects the function of cardiac muscle will affect intrinsic myocardial function (see Table 4.12, point b).

Afterload can be thought of as the work that is demanded of the pump to overcome the resistance to forward flow. If the resistance to flow is low, less work will be required of the pump; if it is high, the pump will have to work harder to produce an equal output. Conditions that alter circulatory resistance (systemic or pulmonary vascular resistance) or cause an obstruction to flow will affect afterload (see Table 4.12, point c). Increases in afterload raise the cardiac oxygen demand, yet there is decreased supply to the subendocardial areas as the contracting muscle squeezes the subendocardial capillaries. If there is a simultaneous tachycardia, the diastolic time interval is reduced and the coronary artery blood flow is reduced, decreasing myocardial oxygen delivery even more.

After surgery, a patient may develop CCF as a result of any of the conditions listed in Table 4.12. Sometimes, multiple factors apply in a single case, and the range of specific disease processes that may produce these problems is wide. Most commonly, it is as a result of fluid overload. The cause of fluid overload may be obvious (*eg* giving blood or parenteral nutrition simultaneously with maintenance fluids to a patient with borderline cardiac function). Fluid balance can also become positive insidiously, perhaps as a result of several days of giving slightly too much maintenance fluid to a small, elderly patient who may also have had routine diuretics omitted or developed atrial fibrillation.

The pathophysiology of CCF is such that the patient enters a downward spiral of increasingly inefficient cardiac function. The physiological response to the failing heart (as it is to surgical pathology) is to increase catecholamine release in an attempt to stimulate cardiac output. Unfortunately, the failing heart has a 'flat Starling curve': one shifted down and to the right compared with the curve in Fig. 4.19. The heart is unable to respond and maintain cardiac output by increasing its stroke volume, and it tends to rely on an increase in rate. This is inefficient in that diastole is short, which reduces the time available for diastolic filling (affecting preload) and for perfusion of the coronary arteries, leading to development of relative or

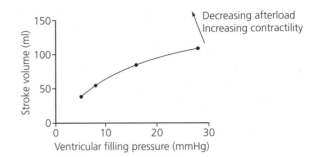

Figure 4.19 *Cardiac function: Starling curve*

absolute ischaemia (and further affecting intrinsic myocardial function).

Cardiogenic pulmonary oedema occurs with acute left ventricular failure or during an exacerbation of congestive cardiac failure. The patient usually has hypertension and ischaemic heart disease and is often elderly. The patient may develop symptoms as a result of MI, or acute ischaemia precipitated by pain from non-cardiac sources. Sudden withdrawal of epidural analgesia may cause acute afterload increases in susceptible patients, while increasing preload as the sympathetic block wears off. The commonest causes are iatrogenic fluid overload, dysrhythmia and MI. Patients become acutely dyspnoeic, orthopnoeic and tachypnoeic. They are tachycardic, sweaty and often hypertensive, and a gallop rhythm may be present with a high JVP. The patient becomes hypoxic with increased work of breathing, which further aggravates myocardial ischaemia. Chest auscultation reveals crepitations basally with some wheeze (cardiac asthma) and, if very severe, pink, frothy sputum may be produced. The CXR may show fluid in the horizontal fissure, peribronchial cuffing, upper lobe diversion, perihilar 'bat's wing' appearance and, rarely, Kerley B lines.

Practice point

Treatment follows ABC principles:

- Give oxygen, sit the patient up and give CPAP as soon as practicable.
- Give diuretics and small doses of opiate intravenously to aid vasodilation, reduce afterload, and decrease anxiety and dyspnoea.
- If intravenous vasodilators/inotropes are considered, transfer to high care area.

The acute management of heart failure is as follows:

- Assess and treat ABCs.
- Give oxygen and monitor SaO_2.
- Stop intravenous infusions (may be only a temporary measure).
- Drugs – consider:
  - diuretics, *eg* furosemide (frusemide) 80 mg i.v.
  - nitrates (patch, sublingual, buccal or i.v.)
  - diamorphine 2.5–5 mg i.v. (but be sure of diagnosis: opiates can kill a patient with acute asthma or chronic bronchitis).
- 12-lead ECG.
- Treat any underlying cause, such as dysrhythmia, pulmonary embolus or tamponade.
- CVP monitoring.
- Early specialist referral.

Cardiogenic shock occurs when there is severe impairment of cardiac function, with hypotension of less than 90 mmHg, or 30 mmHg less than the patient's 'normal' systolic pressure. The patient may be tachycardic or bradycardic. Among the causes (see Table 4.12), the commonest is severe myocardial ischaemia or MI. The cardiac output falls, systemic hypotension occurs and there is a progressive fall in organ perfusion. Left ventricular end diastolic pressure rises and pulmonary venous pressure increases, which leads to pulmonary oedema formation. The patient becomes dyspnoeic and hypoxic, and a downward spiral develops as low SaO_2 and low diastolic pressure further compromise myocardial perfusion. The acutely failing heart is exquisitely sensitive to too much or too little fluid. The patient normally has a high pulmonary artery occlusion (wedge) pressure and pulmonary oedema, so increasing preload with intravenous fluid is often detrimental. Occasionally, the failing heart can have a high preload requirement, and reducing preload by diuresis may worsen cardiac output. If the afterload is high, then reducing it by using vasodilators may be beneficial, but subsequent worsening of hypotension may be detrimental to myocardial perfusion. Accurate individualised treatment requires the measurement of cardiac output, preload and afterload, so invasive monitoring with intra-arterial blood pressure measurement and pulmonary artery catheterisation or transoesophageal Doppler monitoring is required to optimise fluid loading, inotropic support and/or vasodilator therapy. Senior critical care input and monitoring are needed urgently.

Case history 4.2

A 65-year-old woman with longstanding ischaemic heart disease had a right mastectomy two days ago. You are asked to see her on the third postoperative day because she has become acutely short of breath following an episode of severe central chest pain, which lasted about 10 minutes but has since settled.

When you arrive on the ward, the patient is obviously dyspnoeic and is unable to speak in complete sentences. She looks very unwell, and her skin feels cool and clammy. The staff nurse who is with her reports that her pulse rate is 110 bpm and her blood pressure is 170/95 mmHg.

You ask the nurse to give the patient high-flow oxygen, using a mask with a reservoir bag. You examine the patient's chest and find that she has a respiratory rate of 28/min and fine crepitations up to the mid-zones on both sides. It is difficult to hear her heart easily, but you do not think you can hear any murmurs, although you think she has a gallop rhythm. Her blood pressure is now 140/90 mmHg. You ask the nurse to help you sit the patient up and establish intravenous access.

An examination of the patient's ward charts shows that she was progressing well until this episode. The case notes reveal that she is hypertensive, has occasional angina (about one attack every two weeks associated with exercise or cold weather) and usually takes bendroflumethiazide (bendrofluazide) 2.5 mg and atenolol 50 mg each morning. From the prescription, it seems that she has not had these drugs since her operation as she has felt nauseated due to the morphine patient-controlled analgesia she has been using until recently.

Although the patient seems slightly better with the oxygen and repositioning, you decide to give her a dose of furosemide 40 mg intravenously. You ask for an ECG to be obtained and order a CXR. The ECG shows a sinus tachycardia of 100 bpm but is otherwise unchanged from that obtained preoperatively. The CXR confirms pulmonary oedema.

You arrange for the patient to be transferred to the HDU, where she can have continuous ECG, saturation and blood pressure monitoring, and you ask for her to be reviewed by the cardiology team. In the meantime, you arrange for routine blood tests and cardiac enzymes to be sent.

Learning points
- Treat the ABCs first.

- Give high-flow oxygen to all patients during initial assessment.
- Many symptoms can be helped or relieved by repositioning the patient.
- Transfer to a higher level of care when closer monitoring is required.
- Seek expert help early.

Risks of surgery

It is very important to be aware of the risks of surgery in the patient with ischaemic heart disease, particularly the risk of reinfarction (see Table 4.13). It should be evident that delaying surgery, if at all possible, will have a marked effect on the outcome. Unnecessary surgery following an MI may well lead to a case of 'the operation was a success, but the patient died'. Even endoscopy carries some risk.

Table 4.13 *Risk of cardiac disease in non-cardiac surgery*

High risk	Lower risk
MI <6 months	MI >6 months
Unstable angina	Stable angina
Severe aortic stenosis	Abnormal ECG
Decompensated heart failure	Compensated heart failure
Severe hypertension	Compensated valvular lesions
	Cardiac arrhythmias
	Cardiomegaly

The risk of perioperative MI is greater with abdominal and thoracic surgery and is related to the duration of operation.

REINFARCTION RATE
- 60% chance of reinfarction if within three weeks of MI.
- 27% chance if procedure within three months of MI.
- 11% chance if procedure within three to six months of MI.

The presence of cardiac failure preoperatively indicates a significant anaesthetic risk. Measurement of the ejection fraction can help quantify this.

Pulmonary embolism

Pulmonary embolism (PE) is a very important complication that presents in a variety of ways, ranging from immediate death (pulmonary trunk occlusion) to minimal respiratory symptoms or late pulmonary hypertension following multiple small PEs. Many PEs are asymptomatic, and most are preventable by effective deep vein thrombosis (DVT) prophylaxis (see Chapter 9). DVT prophylaxis should start before the operation, but do not forget about patients managed non-operatively.

The clinical effects of embolism depend upon the size of the emboli, whether they are single or multiple, and whether they are acute or chronic. Acute obstruction of the main pulmonary artery causes very severe symptoms, with hypoxia and hypotension due to ventilation–perfusion mismatch and increased right heart afterload, respectively. Small, subsegmental emboli may be clinically insignificant but may herald a further larger embolus from the deep vein source. Clinical diagnosis is difficult, because the most frequent findings – shortness of breath and chest pain – are not specific to PE. The classic combination of dyspnoea, pleuritic chest pain and haemoptysis is very rare. Arterial blood gases may be normal, may show low PaO_2, and may show normal, low or high $PaCO_2$ depending on the severity of the embolus. The only blood test of use is the measurement of D-dimers, which, if normal, effectively excludes PE. It is a waste of time doing this test if the patient has any source of blood clot from another cause (*eg* recent surgery). The CXR is helpful in only about 50% of cases and may show oligaemic lung fields distal to the embolus, pulmonary haemorrhage, local collapse, effusion or diaphragmatic elevation. Again, these changes may be seen in other local chest disease. Transoesophageal echocardiography may show right heart dilation or septal shift to the left or, with large emboli, the embolus itself. A perfusion scan of the lung, if normal, excludes a significant PE. Recent work has suggested that magnetic resonance imaging (MRI) is as sensitive and as specific a diagnostic tool as pulmonary angiography. The ECG is normal in about 50% of cases. Where changes are present, they should not be taken in isolation from the clinical findings. The commonest changes are 'S1, Q3, T3', *ie* large S wave in lead I, large Q wave in V3 and T-wave inversion in lead III, right axis deviation, transient right bundle branch block and T-wave inversion in the right chest leads. These changes are seen in only about 5% of all patients with PE. The larger the PE, the more likely the ECG changes are to occur, but even in massive PE the S1 Q3 T3 syndrome is seen in only about 25% of cases. More often, there are non-specific T-wave changes in the precordial leads and non-specific elevation or depression of the ST segment.

> **Practice point**
>
> - A normal ECG does not exclude the diagnosis of PE.
> - Give oxygen and fluids.
> - CPAP may improve oxygenation.
> - Inotropes will be required if there is hypotension; transfer to high care area.
> - Heparinise or caval filter as indicated.
> - Prevention is better than cure.

Clinical features of PE range from death, through collapse with hypotension (indicating very significant cardiac strain), through pulmonary infarction (often giving rise to the classic signs or pleuritic pain and haemoptysis), to the patient who keeps having 'off days' or who 'fails to progress' as multiple PEs occur.

Diagnosis of PE comes primarily from clinical suspicion. Right heart strain may be reflected in ECG changes (see Table 4.14), elevated JVP or CVP. CXR signs will usually be delayed, and clinical suspicion should be investigated by ventilation–perfusion (V/Q) scanning or pulmonary angiography. If PE is suggested, the patient should also be investigated for sources of further emboli with leg vessel venography or Doppler. Further embolism can be prevented by inserting a caval filter.

Table 4.14 *ECG signs of pulmonary embolism: clinical suspicion is at least as important!*

Tachycardia
Right axis deviation
R wave dominant in V1
Right bundle branch block
S wave in I
T-wave inversion in V1–V3
Q in III
T in III

Patients with cardiovascular compromise may require urgent thrombectomy (by surgical or radiological means) or thrombolysis and should be referred for this. Treatment of less severe emboli will include anticoagulation, which aids the natural thrombolytic processes. Conventional treatment is with continuous intravenous heparin initially followed by long-term (three to six months) warfarin therapy. Recently, low-molecular-weight heparin subcutaneously has become an alternative method of treating emboli in both the short and the long term.

Hypertension

In *chronic hypertension*, avoid stopping long-term antihypertensive medication suddenly, unless the patient is hypotensive. As with almost all cardiac medication, antihypertensive medication should be given on the morning of surgery and reinstituted as quickly as possible afterwards. Many antihypertensive drugs have side effects, including hypokalaemia (diuretics), hyperkalaemia (angiotensin-converting enzyme inhibitors) and impaired responses to hypovolaemia (vasodilators, beta-blockers).

Acute hypertension is often due to pain. Effective analgesia is essential to relieve this, as it puts patients at risk of MI or haemorrhage. Beware of other causes, such as omission of usual antihypertensives, ischaemic heart disease, rupturing aortic aneurysm and other vascular crises, and raised intracranial pressure. Treat any cause and seek expert advice.

Pacemakers

Patients who have pacemakers require surgery not infrequently. Pacemakers can vary between the simple fixed-rate type, although these are used rarely nowadays, to the complex demand type. They can be bipolar or unipolar, the casing acting as the return earth in the case of the latter. It is vital to be aware that your patient has a pacemaker because the use of diathermy can inhibit the demand type; diathermy is less likely to cause problems with a standard fixed-rate type.

Important points to note are:

- Any patient who has a pacemaker and who requires surgery should have had a recent cardiology review to ensure that the pacemaker is functioning optimally.
- Use short rather than long bursts of diathermy.
- The diathermy earthing pad should be placed as far away as possible from the pacemaker, *eg* on the thigh or under the buttocks. Never place the pad on the back of the patient behind the pacemaker.

- Bipolar diathermy is safer than unipolar diathermy.
- Avoid using diathermy near the pacemaker if possible.
- Always monitor the ECG during any procedure.

Pacemaker types are classified using three- or four-letter codes. Classification is based on the chambers that are paced, the response of the pacemaker to a sensed beat and the programmability. Recognition of the codes and details of pacemaker function are beyond the scope of this manual and the CCrISP course. If you have any doubts or worries, contact a cardiologist.

SUMMARY

- The detection and treatment of early clinical signs can prevent major deterioration.
- Abnormal signs must be acted on quickly: patients deteriorate rapidly from cardiovascular problems.
- Normal clinical findings do not always exclude significant abnormality: further investigations and monitoring can help.
- New and longstanding cardiac disorders occur frequently in surgical patients: be aware of common management strategies.
- Impaired perfusion, hypotension, end-organ dysfunction and poor response to treatment suggest severe problems.
- Patients with acute abnormalities of cardiovascular function should not be left without a clear management plan being made, treatment being instituted and a timely reassessment being arranged.
- Higher levels of care are often required, either pre-emptively if the patient has longstanding problems preoperatively or in response to acute events.
- Seek specialist help (anaesthetic/cardiology/ICU) as appropriate at an early stage.

APPENDIX: COMMONLY USED CARDIOVASCULAR DRUGS

Drugs marked *** can be used safely only when the patient is monitored fully on an HDU or ICU. Dosages are given for drugs that can be used rea-

sonably safely outside of the HDU/ICU. Use only drugs with which you are familiar without help from experts.

Antiarrhythmic agents

Amiodarone***

Actions	Prolongs repolarisation of atria and ventricles
Uses	Atrial fibrillation/flutter, ventricular tachycardia
Adverse effects	Hypotension
	Avoid in AV block and with beta-blockers and calcium antagonists
	Thyroid dysfunction: interferes with thyroid function tests. Increases serum levels of digoxin and warfarin

Adenosine***

Actions	Slows conduction through the AV node
Uses	Slows ventricular response in atrial fibrillation/flutter; useful in diagnosing anomalous pathways
	Acts for only 20–30 seconds
Adverse effects	Do NOT use with dipyridamole: prolonged duration of action
	Care with theophylline

Digoxin

Actions	Prolongs AV conduction
	Prolongs depolarisation in atria and has a vagal effect in the SA node
	Positive inotropic effect
	Can cause peripheral vasoconstriction
	Onset of action one to two hours after intravenous administration
Uses	Atrial fibrillation/flutter, heart failure
Adverse effects	Enhanced effect in hypokalaemia, hypomagnesaemia and hypothyroidism
	Do not use in hypertrophic cardiomyopathy, AV block, sick sinus syndrome
Dose	Loading dose 0.2–1.5 mg i.v. or oral in a previously untreated patient

Daily maintenance dose 0.125–0.375 mg

Esmolol***

Actions   Cardioselective beta-blocker
Short-acting: lasts 15–20 minutes
Onset of action two to three minutes
Like other beta-blockers, it prolongs AV conduction, has a negative inotropic effect and can cause peripheral vasodilation

Uses   Atrial fibrillation/flutter

Adverse effects   Hypotension (dose-dependent)
Bronchospasm, especially in asthmatics
Avoid in heart failure, sick sinus syndrome and AV block

Labetalol***

Actions   Combined beta- and alpha-blocker (more beta than alpha effect)

Uses   Hypertension

Adverse effects   Similar to other beta-blockers (compare with esmolol)

Verapamil***

Actions   Calcium channel blocker
Slows conduction in AV node
Coronary artery and peripheral artery vasodilator; less significant effect on systemic and coronary circulation than nifedipine

Uses   Supraventricular tachycardia, atrial flutter/fibrillation

Adverse effects   Hypotension, cardiac failure
Avoid in conjunction with beta-blockers
Increases serum digoxin level
Avoid in Wolff–Parkinson–White syndrome

Lidocaine (lignocaine)

Actions   Membrane stabiliser: suppresses ventricular ectopics and decreases rate of ventricular pacemakers

Uses   Ventricular ectopics

Adverse effects   Convulsions with overdose
Contraindicated in third-degree block with wide QRS complexes

Dose   50–100 mg as bolus dose, followed by infusion of 1–4 mg/min or repeat initial bolus dose at 10 minutes

Magnesium

Uses   Low magnesium may be pro-arrhythmogenic in the critically ill. It is safe to assume that many (if not most) critically ill patients are magnesium-deficient at a cellular level. Common causes of magnesium deficiency include diarrhoea, diuretics, alcohol use and poor dietary intake. Many episodes of atrial fibrillation can be controlled by the administration of magnesium alone

Adverse effects   Magnesium has a wide therapeutic window, but toxic effects include respiratory and cardiac depression, muscular weakness and depression of reflexes

Dose   Loading doses of 10 and 20 mmol i.v. over 15–20 minutes are commonly used, often followed by an infusion to keep the plasma magnesium level at 1–2 mmol/l (usually 40–60 mmol/24 h)

Inotropic agents

Dobutamine

Actions   Stimulation of beta-1 receptors, some effect on beta-2 receptors, slight effect on alpha receptors

Uses   Myocardial failure

Adverse effects   Tachycardia, extrasystoles
May cause hypotension due to beta-2 vasodilator effect; the positive inotropic effect may not be able to compensate for this

Dose   5–10 µg/kg/min intravenous infusion, can be given into a peripheral line

Dopamine

Actions   Stimulation of beta-1 and dopamine receptors
Dose-dependent stimulation of alpha receptors

Uses   Appropriate treatment of shock and/or hypotension
Maintenance of urinary output in low doses; its use for this is controversial, and adequate fluid loading

must be established beyond doubt (CVP line)

Adverse effects Ischaemic necrosis if given via a peripheral line; always administer via a central line

Dose 1–5 µg/kg/min; alpha effect occurs at doses greater than this

Vasoactive agents

Noradrenaline***

Actions Stimulation of alpha receptors and to a lesser extent beta-1 receptors

Marked increase in peripheral resistance with increase in blood pressure and therefore increase in left ventricular afterload

Uses Hypotension in septic shock, but NOT hypovolaemic shock

Adverse effects Constriction of renal vessels, although the increase in blood pressure may partly compensate for any reduction in blood flow

Must be given via a central line.

Glyceryl trinitrate***

Actions Vasodilator; more venous effect in low doses (50 µg/min) with an arterial effect as the dose increases above this, hence reduces preload predominantly in low doses, with a reduction in afterload at higher (arterial) doses

Increases coronary blood flow in ischaemic areas of myocardium

Uses Myocardial ischaemia or MI, heart failure, pulmonary hypertension

Adverse effects Hypotension, avoid in hypovolaemia

Tolerance when given as a continuous infusion for more than about 24 hours

Methaemoglobinaemia in large doses

Objectives

This chapter will help you to:

- Define shock.
- Understand the various aetiologies of shock.
- Recognise the clinical features of a patient with shock.
- Initiate early treatment of the shocked patient.
- Based on the history, clinical condition and response to treatment, decide on an appropriate level of care.

This chapter aims to give a practical clinical overview rather than a detailed account of the pathophysiology of shock. The chapter should be read in conjunction with other chapters, in particular Chapters 2, 4 and 6.

DEFINITION OF SHOCK

> Shock may be defined as acute circulatory failure, with inadequate tissue perfusion causing cellular hypoxia.

Regardless of the underlying cause, shock is characterised by an acute alteration of the circulation in which inadequate perfusion leads to cellular damage, dysfunction and failure of major organ systems.

The clinical features of shock are so variable that they cannot be used to define the shocked state. Although the terms 'hypotension' and 'shock' are often taken to be synonymous, cellular perfusion may be inadequate **despite a normal blood pressure**. Perfusion describes blood flow but also implies the supply of substrates (including oxygen) and the removal of waste products. Use of the term 'inadequate tissue perfusion' rather than 'reduced perfusion' is important since blood flow and substrate supply may be **increased** in hypercatabolic states (*eg* trauma, sepsis) and yet inadequate for the demands of the tissues due to increased metabolism and failure to extract substrates from the circulation (especially in septic shock).

In the shocked state, the **distribution** of blood flow is important. While certain viscera preserve flow through autoregulation (*eg* heart, kidney) others cannot (*eg* skin, gut) and may be hypoperfused preferentially. Intestinal hypoperfusion may occur in the face of a normal pulse and blood pressure, and following a brief hypotensive episode a prolonged period of intestinal hypoxia may occur, with generation of cytokines and the onset of systemic inflammation.

> **Practice point**
> Patients may be in shock despite a normal systolic blood pressure.

AETIOLOGY OF SHOCK

All patients with shock can be regarded as having generalised failure of the circulation. There are four principal categories of shock: hypovolaemic, vasodilatory, cardiogenic and obstructive (see Fig. 5.1 and Table 5.1).

Rapid assessment of the patient may quickly suggest the cause of shock. Keeping in mind this classification helps to avoid the risk of a given diagnosis being overlooked. Of course, the patient may have more than one factor contributing to the shock state, *eg* a patient with abdominal sepsis where the

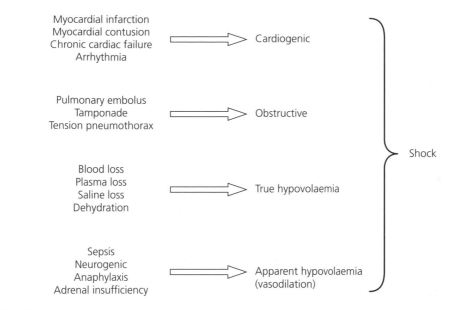

Figure 5.1 *Classification of shock*

primary problem is vasodilation but where hypo-volaemia due to ileus also contributes.

Table 5.1 *Common mechanisms of shock*

Cardiogenic	Pump failure
Hypovolaemic	Fluid loss
Septic	Vasodilation (early)
	Fluid loss (ongoing capillary leak)
	Pump failure (late)
Neurogenic	Vasodilation
Anaphylaxis	Vasodilation and pump failure
Obstructive	Prevents venous return

Hypovolaemic shock

Hypovolaemia is an important cause of low-output shock in which low venous return leads to low car-diac output (see Fig. 5.2). It may result from any of the following causes:

- *Haemorrhage* is a common cause of hypo-volaemia, its effects varying with the duration and severity of blood loss, the patient's age and myocardial condition, and the speed and ade-quacy of resuscitation.
- *Loss of gastrointestinal fluid* may result from vom-iting and diarrhoea, fistulae and sequestration of fluid in the bowel lumen in intestinal obstruction.
- *Trauma and infection* increase capillary perme-

ability, with local sequestration of fluid and oedema. In addition to causing hypovolaemia, trauma and infection may lead to sepsis.

- *Burns* lead to direct loss of fluid from the burned surface and tissue fluid sequestration.
- *Renal loss* of water and electrolytes (*eg* in sodium-losing chronic nephritis, diabetic ketosis or addis-onian crisis) is an occasional cause of shock.
- Frequently, *iatrogenic surgical factors* contribute to hypovolaemia (*eg* poor fluid prescription, slow or tissued intravenous infusion, inappropriate use of diuretics, mechanical bowel preparation, fasting before anaesthesia, insensible fluid losses during prolonged operations and ongoing fluid loss from dissected areas for some hours after surgery).

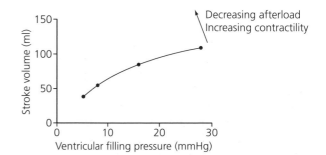

Figure 5.2 *Starling curve plotting ventricular filling pressure (venous return) against stroke volume (cardiac output). The curve is shifted up and to the left by sympathetic stimulation or inotropic agents*

Cardiogenic shock

Primary impairment of cardiac function may result from MI, myocardial ischaemia, acute arrhythmias, acute cardiomyopathy, acute valvular lesions (caused by aortic dissection or trauma) and myocardial contusion.

Obstructive shock

Secondary impairment can result from obstruction to cardiac output, *eg* cardiac tamponade producing constriction of the heart, tension pneumothorax or major pulmonary embolism with obstruction to right ventricular outflow.

In all shock states, myocardial performance is affected adversely by reduced coronary arterial perfusion and in some cases by circulating myocardial depressant substances (*eg* septic shock).

Case history 5.1

You receive a trauma team call to the emergency department: the paramedics have radioed that they will be arriving in four minutes with a 34-year-old patient who has a blood pressure of 80 mmHg systolic and a stab wound to the back between the shoulder blades.

What form of shock might this patient be suffering from:

- haemorrhagic shock?
- pump failure due to pericardial tamponade?
- pump failure due to tension pneumothorax?
- neurogenic shock due to spinal cord transection?

All are possible.

What action may be necessary?
This depends on the cause, but immediate attention to the ABCs, with administration of oxygen and probably fluids, diagnosis and definitive treatment are the mainstays of treatment.

Neurogenic factors

True neurogenic shock follows spinal transection or brainstem injury with loss of sympathetic outflow beneath the level of injury and consequent vasodilation. The rapid increase in size of the vascular bed, including venous capacitance vessels, leads to reduced venous return and reduced cardiac output. There is often a relative bradycardia. An analogous

condition may be seen during epidural analgesia, although in this case the block is seldom high enough to cause a bradycardia.

Anaphylaxis

Anaphylactic reactions are mediated by immunoglobulin E (IgE) antibodies causing massive degranulation of mast cells in sensitised individuals. Activation of mast cells releases histamine and serotonin; with systemic kinin activation, this leads to rapid vasodilation, a fall in systemic vascular resistance (SVR), hypotension, severe bronchospasm, hypoxia and hypercapnia. In contrast to sepsis, the fall in SVR is so sudden and profound that blood pressure falls markedly. Prompt treatment with oxygen, fluids, adrenaline, hydrocortisone and an antihistamine is required. Stop giving the trigger substance!

Endocrine factors

Although adrenal failure is in itself a potent cause of shock (due to the sudden withdrawal of circulating cortisol and aldosterone), the role of the adrenal cortex in the production of shock by other causes is debatable. Acute adrenal failure may occur in severe meningococcal sepsis (Waterhouse–Friderichsen syndrome). Adrenal insufficiency (often subacute) is also seen in patients in whom necessary perioperative steroid cover has been omitted.

Septic shock

Sepsis and septic shock are complex and are covered in more detail in Chapter 7. In septic shock, the patient becomes hypotensive and the tissues are perfused inadequately as a result of organisms, toxins or inflammatory mediators. Common sources include the abdomen, chest, soft tissues, wounds, urine and intravascular lines (central or peripheral) or other medical implants.

CLINICAL FEATURES AND EARLY DIAGNOSIS

It is important to follow a logical sequence in the assessment of potentially shocked patients. A suitable starting point is the ABCs of your immediate management followed by a full patient assessment, including chart review, history, examination and investigations. For a patient on a surgical ward, it is also important to speak to the medical and nursing staff and to note the results of recent investigations. In assessing a patient with shock, some important features to note are:

- Is there an obvious cause that requires immediate treatment?
- Does the age or previous history of the patient suggest a possible myocardial component?
- Has the patient recently received medication that may have an effect on the cardiovascular or respiratory system?
- Does the fluid balance chart of the patient show a gradually deteriorating urine output or likelihood of a significantly abnormal fluid balance? Remember that trends in the charted observations may be more important than absolute values and that patients with hypovolaemic shock may have a normal systolic blood pressure.
- Does the patient have a temperature, high white cell count or a history of an operative procedure that may make sepsis a more likely diagnosis?

The majority of patients with shock have a low cardiac output. An exception is septic shock, in which the cardiac output may be increased. The classic appearance of a patient with low-output shock is that seen after haemorrhage. The features are due partly to loss of circulating volume and partly to intense sympathetic stimulation. In established shock, the patient is pale, with a rapid, thready pulse and cold, clammy extremities. The peripheral veins are collapsed due to reduced filling and sympathetic venoconstriction. The respiratory rate is increased due to chemoreceptor stimulation, and the presence of tachypnoea is an important sign of impending deterioration. The patient becomes restless as a result of cerebral hypoperfusion, and confusion and coma can supervene. Urine output is low (<0.5 ml/kg/h).

In haemorrhagic shock, decreased venous return to the heart results in a low right atrial pressure, low right ventricular end diastolic volume and reduced output. This usually reduces the left atrial and ventricular end diastolic volumes, and stroke volume falls. Since cardiac output (CO=heart rate (HR)×stroke volume (SV)), then, for a fixed SV, an increase in HR is the first compensatory measure available. The only way the body has to increase the SV acutely is to decrease the amount of blood contained in the resistance and capacitance vessels by vasoconstriction, squeezing the periphery to return more blood to the heart. This gives the appearance of the cold, shut-down peripheries. The patient's response to hypovolaemia may be modified in the elderly, in ischaemic heart disease, in patients on beta-blockers, in trained athletes and in young adults.

The effect of haemorrhage on blood pressure is particularly variable. It depends on the duration and magnitude of blood loss, the patient's age and cardiovascular status, and the speed and adequacy of resuscitation. Initially, the systemic blood pressure is maintained; diastolic blood pressure may actually increase, particularly in young patients. Up to 25 or even 30% of circulating volume can be lost without affecting systolic pressure because of the intense vasoconstriction and, to a lesser extent, the shift of fluid from interstitial to intravascular space. A modest further loss (to 35–40% deficit) can precipitate calamitous collapse, perhaps with bradycardia rather than the expected tachycardia.

> **Practice point**
> Systolic blood pressure may be normal in the presence of significant loss of circulating volume.

Early diagnosis

The key to early diagnosis is to look for signs of **decreased tissue perfusion** (see Table 5.2). Capillary refill time can be assessed by observing the return of colour after pressure on the nail beds or earlobes, the presence of cool extremities, or a widening gap between the core and peripheral temperatures, which reflects decreased skin perfusion. A fall in urine output indicates decreased renal per-

Table 5.2 *Signs of decreased tissue perfusion*

Cool peripheries

Poor filling of peripheral veins

Increased respiratory rate

Increased core/peripheral temperature gradient

Capillary refill time prolonged (>2 s)

Poor signal on pulse oximeter

Poor urine output

Restlessness or decreased conscious level

Metabolic acidosis or elevated lactate

fusion, whilst in the absence of a head injury an alteration in conscious level is a useful early sign of decreased cerebral perfusion. In addition, the respiratory rate normally increases before significant tachycardia or hypotension develops. In situations where accurate measurement of blood pressure is possible, an early fall in pulse pressure (difference between systolic and diastolic) reflects the rise in diastolic pressure due to vasoconstriction.

Specific features of cardiogenic shock

Cardiogenic shock shares many of the features associated with haemorrhagic shock. However, whereas the initial treatment of other forms of shock shares common themes, that of cardiogenic shock is very different. Although there is no primary loss of circulating volume, cardiac output falls and catecholamine-induced vasoconstriction still produces cold, clammy extremities. The picture is modified by elevation of cardiac filling pressure leading to elevation of the central or jugular venous pressure and pulmonary oedema.

A careful history and examination of the chest, heart sounds and neck veins together with assessment of a chest X-ray and ECG should prevent the possibility of cardiogenic shock being overlooked in a surgical patient.

Obstructive shock

Cardiac tamponade, tension pneumothorax and pulmonary embolism are the principal causes of obstructive shock. Through a variety of mechanical mechanisms, each mechanically prevents the heart from working well. Typically, the JVP can be elevated in each, and assessment of the JVP should be routine. Tamponade and tension pneumothorax need prompt relief but all can still respond temporarily to intravenous fluids and oxygen.

Specific features of septic shock

Sepsis is dealt with and defined in Chapter 7 and further comments here are limited to the making of a diagnosis. Clearly, haemodynamic instability and pyrexia five to seven days after a colonic resection with anastomosis should be treated with suspicion, but in general the early features of sepsis are subtle

(see Table 5.3), diagnosis is difficult and a high index of suspicion is **essential**. The patient may look remarkably well, due largely to pink, well-perfused extremities. As the patient is already stressed, clues may be obtained from the history or the patient's charts; in postoperative patients, blood gas measurements can aid early diagnosis. A grave error is for inexperienced personnel to treat restlessness (due to hypoxia and hypovolaemia) with sedation rather than appropriate resuscitation.

Table 5.3 *Clinical features of sepsis*

Early	Late
Restlessness and slight confusion	Decreased conscious level
Tachypnoea	Tachypnoea
Tachycardia	Tachycardia
Low SVR	
High cardiac output	Low cardiac output
Systolic BP normal or slightly decreased	Systolic BP <80 mmHg
Oliguria	Oliguria
Metabolic acidosis, elevated blood lactate	Metabolic acidosis, elevated blood lactate
Warm, dry, suffused extremities	Cold extremities

In septic shock, an early effect of the mediators is to cause a fall in SVR due to vasodilation. The decrease in SVR reduces the afterload on the heart and leads to a reflex increase in cardiac output, provided the patient has a healthy myocardium and adequate volume state. Thus, in early sepsis, blood pressure may be well maintained, and often the patient is pink with flushed peripheries and maybe a low diastolic pressure.

In the later stages, or if the patient is already hypovolaemic, the heart may be unable to maintain an adequate output in the face of a falling SVR, so that blood pressure falls (BP = CO × SVR). The patient may then become almost indistinguishable from someone suffering from hypovolaemic shock. Hence, the patient may be hypothermic or hyperthermic, depending on the phase. As the septic process progresses, fluid loss due to increased capillary permeability may also contribute to hypotension, and myocardial depressant factors reduce cardiac function directly. Initially, the patient requires oxygen and fluids, but it is vital that cultures are taken and the source is identified and treated (see Chapter 7).

PRINCIPLES OF MONITORING AND MANAGEMENT

Restoration of adequate perfusion at the cellular level is the essential aim of treatment. In practice, the initial resuscitation of patients with any form of shock is influenced more by the nature of the associated physiological disturbances than by the specific underlying cause. However, the ultimate success of treatment depends largely on detection and elimination of the underlying cause (*eg* arrest of bleeding or drainage of a source of sepsis).

> **Practice point**
> - Resuscitate.
> - Diagnose.
> - Treat the underlying cause.

The mainstays of early treatment are **infusion of fluid** and **oxygen** administration, with the aim of improving cardiac output and oxygen transport. If cardiogenic and obstructive forms of shock can be excluded, then all patients with shock can be treated initially with fluid administration (initial bolus 10 ml/kg crystalloid if normotensive, 20 ml/kg if hypotensive). Oxygen should initially be given in high concentration (12–15 l/min) until blood gas analysis or saturation measurements are available.

Occasionally, you will encounter a patient with major haemorrhage who requires **operative resuscitation**. You will find it very difficult to resuscitate a patient with major haemorrhage, and prolonged attempts are futile and merely lead to coagulopathy, hypothermia and death. Exsanguinating patients need immediate definitive treatment, usually by surgery.

As stressed above, it is the indices of tissue perfusion that are most useful in the early management of hypovolaemia. One should not be misled into thinking that a patient is well perfused simply because the blood pressure and heart rate are normal. On the other hand, a lucid patient with rapid capillary refill, warm, dry skin and a good urine output is unlikely to have significant hypovolaemia.

Monitoring and instrumentation

Successful clinical monitoring depends on the frequent measurement of simple haemodynamic indices and assessment of tissue perfusion, as outlined above. The following guidelines apply to all forms of shock.

VENOUS ACCESS

Good venous access must be obtained early by inserting at least two large-bore (16G) peripheral cannulae. Access is normally obtained in the antecubital fossa or via the cephalic vein at the wrist. If vasoconstriction makes it difficult to gain access, a 'cut-down' can be performed in the antecubital fossa or on the long saphenous vein in front of the medial malleolus. In profoundly shocked patients, it may be necessary to obtain the initial access by cannulating the femoral vein percutaneously in the groin. Draw blood for urgent cross-matching, haematology and biochemistry.

BLADDER CATHETERISATION

A bladder catheter is inserted transurethrally unless there is a possibility of urethral injury (as in severe pelvic fractures) and except when dealing with young children. Under these circumstances, a suprapubic catheter is inserted once the bladder has filled. The urinary catheter is attached to a graduated collecting device (urimeter) so that output can be measured hourly.

ELECTROCARDIOGRAM MONITORING

ECG monitoring will detect arrhythmias and myocardial ischaemia. It is indicated particularly in primary cardiogenic shock, myocardial dysfunction secondary to ischaemia, direct thoracic injury and sepsis. Arrhythmias are more likely when there is electrolyte or acid–base disturbance.

PULSE OXIMETRY

A pulse oximeter attached to a finger or earlobe allows transcutaneous estimation of oxygen saturation of haemoglobin. The accuracy of such peripheral probes depends on good peripheral perfusion. However, in poorly perfused patients, good equipment gives a visual or audible warning of a poor signal, thus providing a useful index of both oxygen transport and tissue perfusion.

CENTRAL VENOUS CATHETERISATION

A catheter can be inserted percutaneously via the internal jugular or subclavian veins so that it lies in the superior vena cava, thus allowing measurement of CVP. In the initial resuscitation of an overtly hypovolaemic patient, time must **not** be wasted inserting a central venous catheter. The small bore and length of the catheter usually prevent rapid infusion, whilst inadvertent damage to the apical pleura during insertion may lead to a pneumothorax, a potentially fatal complication in a patient who is not resuscitated. However, following the initial administration of fluid and oxygen, measurement of CVP can be useful.

In a shocked patient, a low (<5 mmHg) or even negative CVP indicates the need for more fluid. At the other extreme, a very high (>20 mmHg) CVP indicates cardiac failure and the need for diuretics, vasodilators or inotropic agents. In practice, static measurement of CVP can mislead. For example, a young patient may have an apparently normal CVP (say 10 mmHg) as a result of vasoconstriction. A fluid challenge can resolve doubt. This is performed by measuring CVP before and after the administration of a small fluid bolus (100–200 ml). If the CVP does not rise, further fluid can be given safely; a significant rise in CVP suggests myocardial failure or dysfunction and avoids inadvertent overtransfusion. The use of this fluid challenge with CVP measurement can be useful in a ward setting in situations of doubt, but it does not obviate the need for more involved means of cardiac monitoring (such as a pulmonary artery catheter) when the need arises (see Chapter 6).

CORE AND PERIPHERAL TEMPERATURE MEASUREMENT

Using one's own hand to assess skin temperature is useful in shocked patients. If thermistors are used to measure core and peripheral temperatures, the core/peripheral gradient provides a useful index of skin perfusion. Core temperature measurement also detects hypothermia, as in trauma patients who have lain in a cold environment, particularly following water immersion.

Fluid administration

In most cases, the type of fluid lost in shock has little influence on the choice of fluid for initial replace-ment. Successful initial resuscitation depends more on the **rapidity** and **adequacy** of fluid replacement than on the choice of regimen. Initial fluid management consists of boluses of warmed crystalloid (10–20 ml/kg). However, red cell concentrates may be required at an early stage, particularly in injured and/or bleeding patients. Subsequent administration depends on monitoring the **response to treatment**.

CONTINUING ASSESSMENT OF THE SHOCKED PATIENT

- Monitor clinical appearance, noting restlessness and confusion (cerebral hypoxia), respiratory rate and state of the peripheral circulation.
- Monitor pulse rate, systemic blood pressure, hourly urine output and CVP.
- Gain valuable additional information by monitoring or periodically checking:
  - blood urea and electrolyte concentrations
  - haemoglobin concentration, white cell count, haematocrit
  - arterial blood gases
  - blood lactate level
  - pulse oximetry
  - core and peripheral temperature
  - pulmonary capillary wedge pressure.
- Remember to send appropriate samples for bacteriological examination (eg blood, urine, sputum, drain fluids) when sepsis is suspected.
- Most importantly, **diagnose and treat the underlying cause**.

Infusion of large volumes of fluid (of any type, including red cell concentrates) can cause dilution of clotting factors (factors II, V, VII, IX and X and platelets). The resulting coagulopathy may need correction by transfusion of fresh frozen plasma, platelets and cryoprecipitate. This should be done selectively rather than routinely, but a watch must be kept for evidence of coagulopathy. Hospitals usually have guidelines for the use of clotting factors, and you should be aware of these. Considerable degrees of coagulopathy can simply be observed and monitored if active bleeding is not a problem, but clotting factors are needed at an earlier stage if the patient is still bleeding or undergoing surgery. Some synthetic colloids, notably dextrans, can compound coagulopathy. Hypothermia also contributes to bleeding diathesis by causing platelet dysfunction.

Try to ensure that resuscitation fluids are warmed, particularly when massive transfusion is needed.

COLLOID OR CRYSTALLOID?

Synthetic colloids increase circulating volume to a greater degree per volume infused in the short term, but most are redistributed within a few hours in a manner similar to saline. All carry a risk of side effects, notably anaphylaxis and coagulopathy. You should recall to which fluid compartment each fluid type is distributed and also the mechanisms whereby circulating volume is supported by the extracellular and intracellular compartments during hypovolaemic states.

The debate over colloid or crystalloid is well documented. Some of the salient points are:

- In most situations, both types of fluid are able to replenish blood volume if given in sufficient quantity.
- To replace a given amount of blood loss, the volume of crystalloid is approximately three times that of colloid.
- When crystalloid resuscitation is used, there is a greater weight gain and probably more oedema than when colloid is used.
- There is no fixed relationship between serum albumin concentration and colloid osmotic pressure until serum albumin falls below 15 g/l.
- In septic shock with increased capillary permeability, both colloids and crystalloids pass across the vascular basement membrane.
- Colloid can interfere with coagulation under some circumstances.
- Many experienced practitioners limit the volume of colloid used during resuscitation to <50% of non-blood fluid or 1–1.5 l, whichever is the lesser.

More importantly, the principal changes in practice that occur with experience are the early identification and rapid treatment of hypovolaemic states, a prompt utilization of blood when haemorrhage is occurring and, most importantly, the surgical treatment of any **underlying cause**, particularly haemorrhage.

Refractory shock

If hypovolaemic shock proves refractory to fluid replacement and oxygen administration, then the factors shown in Table 5.4 may be responsible.

Table 5.4 *Refractory shock*

Underestimation of the degree of hypovolaemia
Failure to arrest haemorrhage
Presence of cardiac tamponade or tension pneumothorax
Underlying sepsis
Secondary cardiovascular effects due to delay in instituting treatment
Further action is necessary!

Assessment of response

One of the most important steps in the management of the shocked patient is the assessment of the response to treatment. For every exsanguination, you will meet many more patients who become critically ill with shock in a less dramatic but no less important manner. During resuscitation and no more than every 30 minutes or so, you should reassess the patient's progress. If the signs are not improving, then you need to change your plan of action (see Table 5.5). The aim is to detect those patients whom you have initially misjudged and those who are temporary responders. Such patients are common, and it can be difficult to assess the need for surgery. Involve senior help if you are in doubt.

Table 5.5 *Response to treatment of shock*

No response, eg exsanguination
Temporary response, eg continuing slow but steady postoperative haemorrhage
Full response, eg simple sepsis caused by repeat urinary catheterisation, which responds to resuscitation and antibiotics

Algorithm of cardiovascular monitoring/support

See Table 5.6.

Many surgical patients become hypovolaemic and present with oliguria, hypotension, tachycardia, hypoxia or acidosis in isolation or almost any combination. Many do not develop a full picture of shock but require prompt treatment just the same. Most are treated simply with conventional measures, including adequate fluid replacement (and other necessary treatments). You need to have a method of management clear in your mind. You should review

Table 5.6 *Algorithm of cardiovascular monitoring/support*

1 Establish and maintain normovolaemia:

Assess with CCrISP system

Give reasonable intravenous fluid challenge (10–20 ml/kg crystalloid initially, see text)

Treat any underlying cause (blood loss, sepsis, etc)

Determine recent fluid balance

2 Assess response:

Clinically (perfusion, BP, urine output, JVP, pulse)

By simple investigations (repeat full blood count (FBC), pulse oximetry, pH, base excess)

Improving?

Adjust fluid regimen

Treat underlying cause

Plan to review shortly

Deteriorating?

Resuscitate and involve expert help directly

No progress?

Reassess:

?different diagnosis: treat and seek help

?still hypovolaemic: continue fluids and find/treat cause

Not sure if normovolaemic

Insert CVP

3 CVP

Inadequate? Establish normovolaemia

Adequate (>8 cmH₂O) but inadequate circulation?

Reassess cause (and treat as necessary)

Consider inotrope (if permitted by local protocol and if qualified)

No/poor response: seek help directly

High (>15 cmH₂O) and patient exhibits signs of cardiac failure

Simple left ventricular failure (LVF): treat

Suspect cardiogenic shock: call for help

4 Arterial, PA catheterisation and inotrope treatment: transfer to ICU

the patient later to ensure that normal function has definitely been re-established. Patients who need anything more than simple correction of minor to modest fluid deficit should be managed in a high-dependency environment. There is no point inserting monitoring lines when the staff do not have both the knowledge and the time to make use of them.

Remember to treat any underlying pathology, particularly haemorrhage (which often needs surgery), in addition to giving intravenous fluids and oxygen.

Patients who have incipient failure of more than one system need the help of an intensivist directly. In any event, you should have a very low threshold

for involving help and informing your consultant. All these patients should be receiving monitored oxygen therapy.

Young and fit patients tolerate rapid infusion well, and CVP insertion is indicated when there is doubt about progress, adequacy of filling or likely tolerance of the administered fluid.

Patients who continue with inadequate cardiovascular function and in whom good cardiovascular filling has been confirmed by CVP measurement may require inotropic support. In these cases senior help should be mandatory and patients should be treated in a critical care environment. In some units, local protocols may allow administration of a single inotrope outside the ICU, but these should be administered cautiously with a low threshold for transfer to the ICU, with whom the case should already have been discussed.

Metabolic monitoring in refractory shock

Urea and electrolyte levels are required to establish a baseline and monitor progress. Arterial pH and blood gas measurements are essential to assess hypoxia, hypercapnia and acid–base balance. Blood lactate levels are a good index of cellular hypoxia and hepatic function.

Metabolic acidosis associated with inadequate perfusion will correct rapidly once cardiac output is improved; indeed, its disappearance is a marker of adequate resuscitation. It is rarely necessary to give bicarbonate.

Respiratory acidosis with an increase in arterial PaCO₂ usually indicates the need for endotracheal intubation and assisted ventilation.

Higher levels of care

Shock is an immediately life-threatening condition and demands treatment as such. The ability of the CVS to compensate has been discussed, and shock reflects the state that is reached once decompensation is occurring. While uncomplicated hypovolaemia can often be managed satisfactorily without intensive care facilities, patients with severe trauma, sepsis, cardiogenic shock or shock complicated by secondary myocardial dysfunction will all benefit from the monitoring and support available in an ICU. Consideration should be given to early ICU admission for patients with significant comorbidity, since an ICU can then play a prophylactic role. Similarly, patients who fail to respond quickly and completely should be discussed with the ICU and a surgical consultant. Assessment and monitoring of the CVS are detailed in Chapter 6. The basis of ICU care is the same as outlined previously, with attention to fluid administration, oxygenation and definitive treatment.

Based on the underlying cause of shock and measurement of cardiovascular parameters (particularly the confirmation of an adequate circulatory volume), some patients require inotropic support. The selection of an inotropic agent is based on the cardiovascular effects of the drug and the underlying pathophysiology. The cardiovascular effects of many agents can be predicted from a knowledge of their particular effect on adrenergic receptors (see Table 5.7). Their effect on cardiac function is shown in Fig. 5.2.

SUMMARY

- *Definition:* acute circulatory failure, with inadequate tissue perfusion causing cellular hypoxia.
- *Diagnosis:*
  - assess perfusion and not simply blood pressure; and
  - identify the different patterns.
- *Treatment:*
  - restore perfusion;
  - common initial approach with oxygen and fluids, except for cardiogenic shock;
  - treat the underlying cause; and
  - determine the appropriate level of care.

Table 5.7 *Action of inotropic agents*

Drug	Receptor action	Effect	Clinical use
Noradrenaline	Alpha-adrenoceptor agonist	Vasoconstriction	Septic shock with low SVR
Adrenaline	Alpha and beta agonist (predominantly beta-1)	Positive inotropic and chronotrope Vasoconstriction	Widespread in conditions of low cardiac output
Dopamine	Dopamine receptor agonist Alpha and beta agonist	Low dose: increased renal and hepatic blood flow, splanchnic vasodilation	Used as first-choice inotrope on some ICUs for its inoconstrictor effects. Not commonly used at low doses
		Medium dose: beta 1 effects causing tachycardia and increased contractility	
		High dose: alpha effects causing vasoconstriction	
Dobutamine	Beta-1 and beta-2 agonist	Increases cardiac output and reduces SVR	Cardiogenic shock (used in coronary care units)
Dopexamine	Dopamine receptor agonist	Increases splanchnic blood flow	Limited proven use

Cardiovascular monitoring 6
and support

Objectives

This chapter will help you to:

- Understand the indications for invasive monitoring.
- Be familiar with the methods used.
- Be aware of the limitations and complications of monitoring.
- Understand how drug and fluid therapy may be used to manipulate cardiovascular function.

This chapter does not intend primarily to teach the practical procedures for insertion of the various lines used for invasive monitoring. This is best learned by practical instruction during the CCrISP course or from an experienced practitioner. Outlines of the techniques are given here.

INTRODUCTION

In the majority of patients, evaluation of cardiovascular function can be achieved by history, examination, measurement of urine output and basic investigations. These will provide information on how well the CVS is fulfilling its basic function of delivering oxygen and nutrients to the tissues and removing carbon dioxide and other products of tissue metabolism. The efficacy of the system in achieving this goal depends upon the production of a cardiac output sufficient to meet the demands of tissue metabolism over a wide range in both health and disease and ensuring that the regional distribution of the cardiac output is matched to the metabolic needs of individual organs (see Table 6.1).

Table 6.1 *Determinants of cardiac output*

Preload	Filling pressure
Cardiac function	Rate, rhythm, contractility
Afterload	Total peripheral resistance

In critically ill patients, deviation from the normal ranges of any of these components of cardiac output can occur unexpectedly, rapidly and with little to see clinically in the early stages of cardiovascular deterioration. Objective measurements showing change should be detected as early as possible to allow rapid corrective therapy before organ damage has occurred. Modern monitoring equipment can provide rapid, accurate and reproducible measurements of cardiovascular performance and the effects of treatment.

Cardiovascular therapy in the critically ill aims to avoid tissue hypoxia. The degree to which one must go to monitor the adequacy of the CVS in achieving this goal varies with severity of illness and complexity of the case. Organs vary in their ability to maintain their own perfusion (through autoregulation) and, generally, measurements relate the total body picture rather than adequacy of perfusion of specific viscera. Certain organs, notably the gut, are prone to hypoxia, which may continue to drive the inflammatory process (including multiple organ failure) even once the initial causal factors have been dealt with. To overcome this, one approach has been to try to ensure that the critically ill patient with multiple organ failure has a circulation that provides an oxygen delivery that is, if anything, greater than normal, thus minimising the chance of occult hypoxia. A related approach has been to monitor plasma lactate level and/or negative base excess on the grounds that elevated values of these suggest that tissue hypoxia may be present. An alternative strategy is to try to measure specific visceral perfusion in suspect viscera (such as the intestine) by techniques such as tonometry. There is much to be said for pursuing similar objectives, at an appropriate level, in all unwell patients, and particularly in the preoperative preparation of the critically ill surgical patient.

In broad terms, the indications for invasive monitoring of the cardiovascular system are:

- failure to promptly restore and maintain cardiovascular homeostasis with simple techniques (intravenous fluids, surgery, non-invasive blood pressure, pulse oximetry);
- during procedures that may give rise to rapid or profound changes in preload or afterload;
- during treatment with vasoactive drugs that influence preload, afterload or myocardial function; and
- in any patient who has, or is at risk of developing, a low perfusion state from any cause.

The parameters that can be monitored include:

- *intra-arterial blood pressure:* systolic, mean and diastolic;
- *CVP*, indicating preload of pulmonary circulation and a rough guide to systemic preload given a number of provisos;
- *pulmonary artery pressure (PAP):* systolic, mean and diastolic;
- *pulmonary artery occlusion or 'wedge' pressure (PAOP),* indicating the preload of the systemic circulation; and
- *cardiac output (CO) or cardiac index (CI):* indexing corrects any variable for patient size.

TRANSDUCERS

While the physical principles of how these individual measurements are made are beyond the scope of this course, certain basic scientific principles apply. Changes in any parameter to be measured must be detected accurately with sufficient sensitivity, over the range required, at a suitable frequency response, often from inaccessible sites, and converted by a transducer so that the signals vary in proportion to the changes in the parameters under study. A transducer converts the mechanical energy of pressure changes to electrical energy in a manner such that the electrical output of the transducer varies directly with the change in pressure. An example of this kind of system is shown in Fig. 6.1.

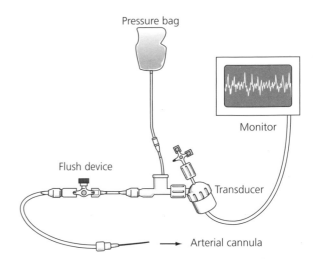

Figure 6.1 *Signal conduction from an arterial cannula. The pressure wave is transmitted from the artery (in this case) to the transducer through relatively rigid tubing. The transducer converts the mechanical signal to an electronic one, displayed on the monitor. The three-way tap on the transducer allows zeroing. Patency of the cannula is maintained by a slow constant flush of heparinised saline under pressure, and most systems incorporate a button for bolus flushing to clear any debris and improve the signal*

The electrical signals must be displayed and processed so that derived results may be calculated. The measurement system must be zeroed and calibrated. If pressure is measured, this should be done with the transducer level relative to the point within the patient at which the pressure is to be measured. Care should be taken to minimise the interference and damping of the measurement signal to ensure an optimal signal-to-noise ratio. Failure to zero or calibrate will produce erroneous results. This can also happen when the cannula or catheter is kinked, abuts the vessel wall or is partly occluded by clot.

SAFEGUARDS

Before considering the individual techniques, one should be aware of certain ground rules common to all procedures used during invasive monitoring methods:

- A sound knowledge of relevant practical anatomy is required.
- Competency in the technique of insertion of the line is required.

- The procedure should be explained to the patient.
- All procedures must be performed using aseptic technique.
- Contraindications and complications must be known.
- The benefit accrued must exceed the risks of the procedure.
- The patient must be in the care of people who know how to manage the lines, all of which must be Luer-locked to prevent disconnection.
- All lines should be labelled clearly, and injections into/sampling from lines should be performed *only* at designated sites.
- Attendants should be familiar with the monitors to ensure that the data derived from them is accurate.
- Lines must be dressed aseptically and changed at appropriate intervals.

ARTERIAL ACCESS

This involves cannulation of a peripheral artery either to allow beat-to-beat measurement of arterial blood pressure by connecting the cannula to a transducer or to allow for repeated sampling of arterial blood for analysis. The radial artery and the dorsalis pedis are the most commonly used sites using 20 or 22G sized cannulae. The brachial and femoral arteries should be avoided if possible because of lack of collaterals and, in the case of the femoral site, the risk of sepsis.

When using the radial artery, always check for ulnar flow (*eg* by using Allen's test) before cannulation (see Fig. 6.2). Local sepsis and coagulopathy are the main contraindications. Complications include haematoma, thrombosis, distal ischaemia, intimal damage, aneurysm formation, disconnection and injection of irritant drugs. Samples from arterial cannulae should be taken aseptically and the line flushed and resealed afterwards. After cannulation of the artery, the cannula should be connected to a continuous flush device containing heparinised saline under pressure, which maintains patency and allows blood pressure changes to be conducted without letting blood flow out of the artery into the line (see Fig. 6.3).

If measurement of pressure is the goal, then the arterial cannula is connected via a relatively short length of rigid line to a three-way tap, flush device

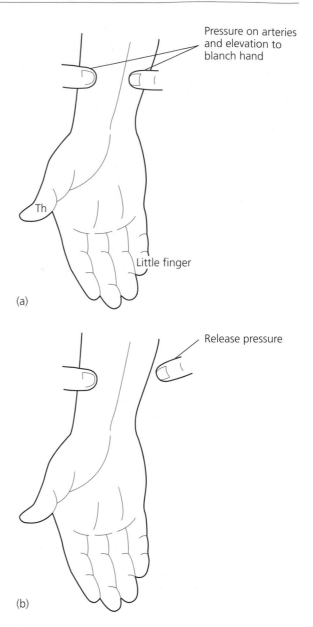

(a)

(b)

Figure 6.2 *Allen's test. Blanch the hand by clenching the fist, then simultaneously occlude the radial and ulnar arteries at the wrist. An adequate pink flush of the hand on release of the ulnar pressure confirms an adequate ulnar supply to the palmar arterial arches*

and transducer. Check that the transducer is zeroed and calibrated at the correct level and that the lines contain no air bubbles, which would cause damping of the signal. The shape of the pressure waveform can sometimes reflect the presence of hypovolaemia, when a sharp peaked upswing and downswing with a low dicrotic notch is seen, but it is dangerous to

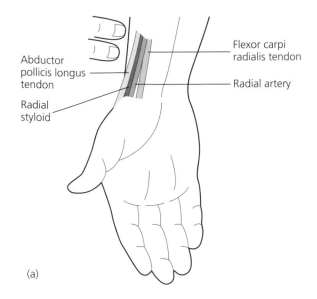

Abductor pollicis longus tendon

Radial styloid

Flexor carpi radialis tendon

Radial artery

(a)

Figure 6.3 *Site for radial arterial cannulation/puncture:*

- *Position the hand and yourself comfortably, with adequate light and assistance.*
- *Palpate the artery with two fingers.*
- *Feel and imagine its course above and below the point of entry.*
- *Insert at 45 degrees, avoiding the superficial vein that often overlies.*

Puncture:

- *Advance the needle tip in a linear fashion. Do NOT wiggle it around!*
- *If you miss, repalpate and search in a systematic fashion with further straight insertions.*
- *Let the syringe fill and withdraw.*
- *Pressure haemostasis: five minutes.*

Cannulation:

- *Puncture as above.*
- *Advance the guidewire.*
- *Railroad the cannula.*
- *Check the backflow and secure the cannula.*
- *Connect the transducer and flushing set-up.*

(b)

Puncture
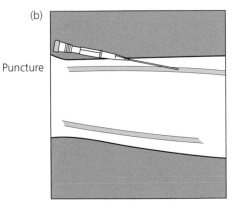

Advance guidewire
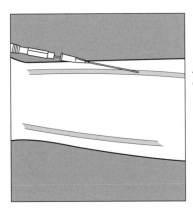

Railroad cannulation
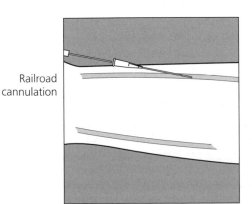

Connect and secure
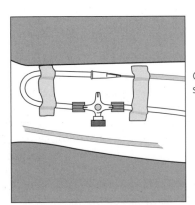

draw such conclusions unless the system is damped adequately (see Fig. 6.4).

CENTRAL VENOUS PRESSURE MEASUREMENT

CVP is simply the pressure within the superior vena cava (SVC) as it enters the right atrium. The best zero reference point visible on the surface of the body is the mid-axillary line. The alternative, the second intercostal space at the sternal edge, represents a point about 5 cm above the atrium. For readings to be comparable at separate times, they should always be taken with the patient supine and from the same point. The pressure may be measured using either a liquid manometer filled with sterile dextrose 5% or by an electronic transducer reading over a suitable pressure range in centimetres of water (see Fig. 6.5).

The 'water' manometer is cheap, effective and simple and can be used on ordinary wards, but it does not respond to rapid changes in pressure. Its response time is, however, sufficiently fast to show the fluctuation in CVP with inspiration (fall in pressure) and expiration (rise in pressure), a change that confirms that the manometer is reflecting the normal change in CVP with fluctuation of intrathoracic pressure. The electronic transducer is faster, and the analysis of the signal produced allows the mean pressure to be displayed, taking into account the variation with the respiratory cycle. The set-up of the transducer is identical to that for arterial pressure measurement, except that the transducer has a range and calibration in centimetres of water rather than millimetres of mercury.

Indications for central venous pressure measurement

- Fluid replacement during therapy for hypovolaemia when conventional access is not possible

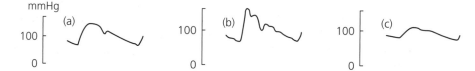

Figure 6.4 Arterial waveforms showing influence of damping: (a) adequately damped; (b) underdamped; (c) overdamped

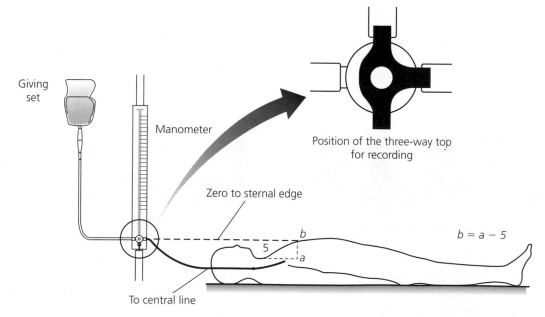

Figure 6.5 Liquid manometer for CVP

or when concern exists about over-transfusion. *Central vein cannulation is NOT advocated as a primary route of access.*

- To measure the effect of vasoactive drugs, particularly vasodilators, on venous capacitance.
- To aid diagnosis of right ventricular failure, when a high pressure will be seen in the presence of poor cardiac output.

> Remember: CVP does not 'equal' intravascular volume and is not an indicator of left ventricular function.

Pitfalls in practice

- *Inaccurate readings* as a result of failure of zeroing or calibration, placement of the cannula tip in the right ventricle, tricuspid regurgitation and incompetence with a large reflux pressure wave, giant 'a' waves, AV dissociation and nodal rhythms.
- *Variations* in intravascular volume, sympathetic tone, cardiac output and intrathoracic pressure (particularly during positive pressure ventilation) may lead to a false impression of a much higher right ventricular filling pressure than is actually present (see Fig. 6.6).
- *Complications* of central line insertion are numerous and relate to damage to the veins themselves and adjacent structures. Complications include rupture of vessel and haemorrhage with local haematoma or haemothorax, tension pneumothorax (particularly if the patient is on positive-pressure ventilation), air embolism, extravascular catheter placement, knotting of catheters, catheter breakage, catheter misplacement, neurapraxia, arterial puncture, lymphatic puncture, tracheobronchial puncture and, most importantly, sepsis.
- The route for access to the central venous circulation depends on the *skill and experience* of the operator and the presence of site-specific contraindications, such as local sepsis, coagulopathy, abnormal anatomy, operative site and previous vein usage (see Fig. 6.7).
- *Before* using the line and acting on measurements made, always check for easy aspiration of blood, pressure fluctuation with respiration and confirmation of position on X-ray.

The UK National Institute for Clinical Excellence (NICE) recommends that two-dimensional ultrasound imaging should be used to guide placement of central venous catheters into the internal jugular vein in elective situations. NICE recommends further that all those involved in placing central venous catheters should undertake training to achieve competence in the use of ultrasound for this purpose. Ideally, ultrasound should be used in either elective or emergency cases if the practitioner is skilled in its use. The anatomical landmark method is still recommended for the subclavian route.

PULMONARY ARTERY CATHETERISATION

Pulmonary artery balloon flotation catheters, also called Swann–Ganz or PA catheters, are multilumen catheters with an inflatable balloon just proximal to the tip. There are usually at least three lumina: one to inflate the balloon with air, one to measure pressure from the catheter tip, and one to measure pressure from the SVC or right atrium and to allow injection or infusion of drugs. Within the catheter wall are thermistors to detect temperature changes and, in some types of modern catheter, coiled-wire heating elements to generate changes in temperature. Pressure can be transduced from the central veins, right atrium, right ventricle and pulmonary artery as the catheter passes through these structures. When placed correctly in a central vein, inflation of the balloon results in the tip of the catheter being carried in the direction of the maximal blood flow as the catheter is fed onwards. Transducing the pressure

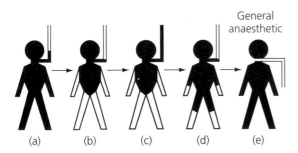

General anaesthetic

(a)   (b)   (c)   (d)   (e)

Figure 6.6 *CVP and intravascular volume: pitfalls in the shocked surgical patient. (a) Normal; (b) shocked but compensating (by peripheral vasoconstriction) with low CVP; (c) rapid refill and (temporarily) high CVP; (d) redistribution and falling CVP as degree of compensatory vasoconstriction lessens; (e) general anaesthesia with vasodilation, loss of compensation and very low CVP*

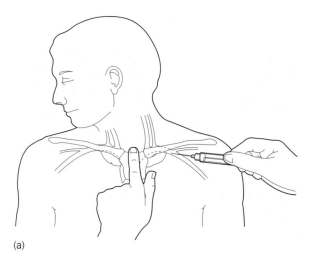

(a)

Figure 6.7 *(a) Central vein cannulation: infraclavicular subclavian route*

- *Tilt the patient 20 degrees head down, arms by the side and head turned away from the side of entry.*
- *Make a skin nick and insert the cannula 1–2 cm below the midpoint of the clavicle.*
- *Advance horizontally towards the suprasternal notch: remember, advance the needle tip in a linear fashion – do NOT wiggle it around!*
- *Try to visualise the anatomy beneath as you do the procedure: think where your needle tip is, particularly in relation to the clavicle and pleura, and the narrow gap between the clavicle and the first rib, where the subclavian artery and vein run.*
- *If you miss, search in a systematic fashion with further straight insertions, trying to picture where the vein is most likely to be.*
- *When venous blood is aspirated freely, remove the syringe and insert the guidewire.*
- *Leave enough guidewire outside to let you railroad the catheter over it without losing the wire inside the patient.*
- *Advance the catheter to a previously measured point, so the tip lies in the distal SVC.*
- *Secure the catheter and check its position by CXR.*

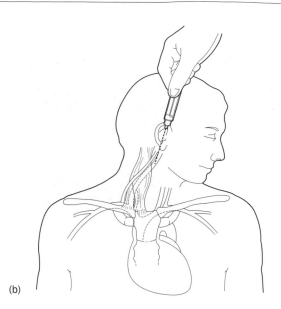

(b)

Figure 6.7 *(b) Central vein cannulation: internal jugular venous route*

- *Try to palpate the vein at the medial border of sternomastoid, at the level of the thyroid cartilage, and imagine its course anterolateral to the carotid artery.*
- *Displace the artery medially and advance the needle through a skin nick.*
- *Advance inferiorly at 30 degrees to the skin, parallel to the artery but lateral. This is often towards the ipsilateral nipple.*
- *Puncture and proceed as above.*
- *Pneumothorax is less likely but still possible with this route.*
- *You should learn and practise one route initially: your anaesthetist will be glad to teach you.*

from its tip allows the position of the catheter to be followed through the right heart into the pulmonary artery, until the decreasing diameter of the pulmonary artery lumen halts its progress and it becomes 'wedged' (see Fig. 6.8).

When wedged, the tip of the catheter beyond the balloon is sealed off from arterial pulsation by the balloon and measurements of pressure made from the tip will reflect the pressure within the vessel lumen distal to this point (see Fig. 6.8). This is known as the PAOP or pulmonary capillary wedge pressure (PCWP). The continuous column of blood from this point extends to the left atrium (there are no valves in the pulmonary circulation) and consequently it is an index of left atrial pressure (LAP). LAP reflects left ventricular end diastolic pressure

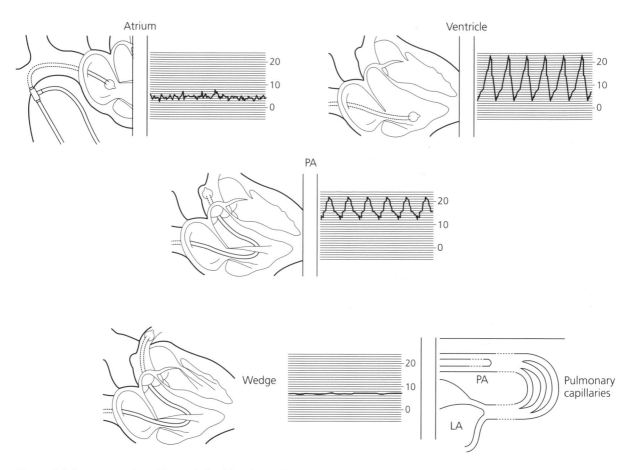

Figure 6.8 *Pressures and waveforms during PA catheter placement*

(LVEDP), which in turn reflects left ventricular end diastolic volume (LVEDV), the true preload. This presupposes normal left ventricular compliance and normal mitral valve function. Changes in PAOP should thus reflect changes in intravascular volume, filling pressure and left ventricular function.

Cardiac output can be calculated using a thermodilution technique in which a known volume of cold saline at a known temperature is injected at a fixed rate via the injectate port of the catheter into the blood of the right atrium, the temperature of which is also known. As the blood and injectate mix on passage through the right ventricle into the pulmonary artery, a small drop in temperature occurs, which is proportional to the cardiac output. A similar calculation can be made if the blood is heated and cooled over a fixed distance and timescale using

'continuous' cardiac output catheters. If the values are divided by the body surface area (BSA), then a CI is produced that eliminates the effect of body size, thus providing more manageable normal ranges.

Having measured CVP, PAOP, CI, BSA, heart rate and mean arterial pressure and taken blood samples from the tip of the catheter, it is possible to calculate a number of derived variables that give further information of great use in the clinical management of complicated cases such as myocardial dysfunction, SIRS/sepsis and acute respiratory distress syndrome (ARDS) (see below). Many of the drugs used to control the CVS in organ failure have competing actions, and their net function cannot always be determined in an individual without the assistance of these techniques.

VARIABLES DERIVED FROM PA CATHETER MEASUREMENTS

- Systemic vascular resistance (SVR):
  - if too high (vasoconstriction), then tissue hypoperfusion is likely
  - if too low, then maintenance of an adequate mean blood pressure will be difficult
- Pulmonary vascular resistance (PVR)
- Stroke volume (SV), stroke index (SI): major determinant of cardiac output and governable by preload
- Left ventricular stroke work index (LVSWI): index of the function of the systemic side of the heart
- Oxygen delivery (DO_2): index of the oxygen delivered to all tissues
- Oxygen uptake (VO_2): index of oxygen consumption

Some of these derived variables are related more closely to vital cardiovascular function and outcome than blood pressure and CVP. Some intensivists maximise VO_2 on the understanding that, until maximal values are reached, occult tissue hypoxia must be present. Controversy exists over the extent to which this goal should be pursued.

Table 6.2 *Indications for pulmonary artery catheterisation*

Preoperatively in high-risk surgical patients, *eg* recent MI or severe CVS disease

Postoperative MI or cardiogenic shock

Any patient requiring infusion of vasoactive drugs to manipulate preload, afterload or oxygen transport

To assist in fluid management in multi-trauma, massive blood loss, SIRS/sepsis and multiple organ failure

Diagnosis of non-cardiogenic pulmonary oedema, as in ARDS

Complications of pulmonary artery catheterisation

PA catheters need to be inserted via large-bore, valved introducers inserted into large central veins, usually the internal jugular or subclavian. As a result, many of the potential complications are those that you would find from central venous cannulation itself. In addition, technique-specific complications include:

- atrial and ventricular dysrhythmias during insertion;
- valvular erosion, sterile or infected valvular vegetations;

- pulmonary embolus, infarction or rupture of pulmonary artery;
- knotting of the catheter within the heart; and
- infection, haematoma or thrombosis at the site of insertion.

Pitfalls in practice

Before acting on the results obtained, you must be sure of their accuracy. Specific problems include:

- Correct catheter placement should be confirmed by CXR, PAOP < mean PAP, wedged PaO_2 > mixed venous PaO_2, and the catheter should flush easily when wedged.
- The tip of the catheter should be in a zone of pulmonary vasculature where the pulmonary capillary pressure is always greater than alveolar pressure in order to ensure continuity between the pressure measured from the tip of the catheter and the left atrium (LA).
- High intrathoracic pressure will introduce an artefact elevating PAOP by 1 mmHg for each 5 cm of PEEP applied during ventilation, although a greater inaccuracy occurs if the patient is hypovolaemic or if the catheter tip is in a zone of low pulmonary blood flow.
- Mitral regurgitation gives a falsely high PAOP as a result of the large 'v' wave produced. A reading from the top of the 'a' wave reflects LAP more accurately.
- The catheter may 'migrate' and produce a wedged trace when the balloon is deflated. If so, it must be withdrawn until the PA trace is visible, otherwise prolonged wedging will produce distal pulmonary infarction.
- Never leave the balloon inflated after completing the PAOP measurement, and always allow it to deflate passively. Never withdraw the catheter with the balloon inflated, as this may cause vascular rupture.

Never insert a PA catheter unless the benefit to the patient outweighs the risk of the procedure.

NON-INVASIVE MEASUREMENT OF CARDIAC FUNCTION

Some studies have shown increased morbidity and mortality in patients who had PA catheters inserted. This has created controversy and resulted in non-invasive methods of measurement being developed. There are several techniques, among which transoesophageal Doppler (TOD) and pulse contour cardiac output with indicator dilution (PiCCO) are used most widely. Such techniques cannot wholly replace PA catheters, since they do not provide direct pressure measurements.

TOD uses the Doppler shift principle to make measurements of blood velocity in the descending aorta. A disposable Doppler probe contained at the tip of a $90\,cm \times 5.5\,mm$ probe is passed down the oesophagus to lie at the level of the descending aorta (around 35–45 cm) and rotated until a triangular arterial waveform is displayed as the shift signal is displayed as a velocity/time plot. The shape of the waveform provides information on preload, stoke volume and afterload (see Fig. 6.9). The area under the curve represents the stroke volume flowing through the descending aorta; applying a factor determined from the patient's age, height and weight allows the stroke volume to be calculated. A number termed the corrected flow time (FTc) is calculated: this is low in hypovolaemia and may be used to derive the SVR index (SVRI). The disadvantage of the TOD is that the patient must be anaesthetised and intubated to tolerate the probe. It cannot be used in patients who have coarctation of the aorta or who are on intra-aortic balloon pumps.

PiCCO calculates cardiac output from a peripheral arterial cannula that feeds beat-to-beat information to a computer, which follows the heart rate and pressure waveform and integrates the area under the curve. The accuracy of the method is improved as the cannula also contains a sensitive thermistor to detect the small drop in the temperature of arterial blood that follows the injection of a bolus of ice-cold saline into a central vein. This change in blood temperature is proportional to cardiac output, a process known as thermodilution. PiCCO is calibrated automatically each time a thermodilution is performed.

CARDIOVASCULAR SUPPORT USING VASOACTIVE DRUGS

In the normal heart, cardiac output is determined by preload, afterload, heart rate, rhythm, contractility, and balance of oxygen demand and supply. If the heart is damaged, then, for a given preload or afterload, cardiac output will decrease. This can be represented graphically either by pressure/volume loops or by the more familiar Starling curve (see Fig. 4.19 in Chapter 4).

Invasive cardiovascular monitoring collects data that allow the construction of such curves so that the effects of varying preload, afterload, inotropes, etc, can be recorded accurately, ensuring that therapy is producing an objective improvement in the patient's cardiovascular status. However, the curves are time-consuming to plot and often adjustments to fluid loading, vasodilation and inotropic support are made on the basis of CI measurements primarily.

If the CI remains low after correcting any hypovolaemia with a fluid challenge, then inotropic or other vasoactive drugs are used with the aim of optimising myocardial contractility by balancing myocardial oxygen supply and demand. Accurate measurements of derived variables can predict probable therapeutic regimens (see Table 6.3).

Drugs that increase cardiac output and ejection fraction are known as inotropes. Ideally, in addition to these properties, they should reduce afterload and preload, resulting in decreased transventricular wall tension, promoting coronary blood flow, increasing myocardial oxygen delivery and reducing oxygen consumption. Regrettably, the ideal inotrope does not exist, but the most commonly used are adrenaline, noradrenaline and dobutamine. They all act by providing an upward left shift in the Starling curve, as shown in Fig. 4.19 in Chapter 4.

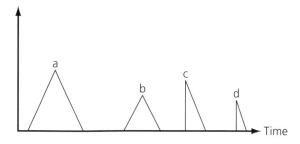

Figure 6.9 *Stylised TOD waveforms for vascular abnormality. (a) Best waveform: normal configuration. (b) Failing left ventricle: decreased waveform height and low peak velocity. Giving inotropes increases waveform height and restores velocity. (c) Hypervolaemia: narrow waveform base with decreased corrected flow time (FTc). Giving volume lengthens flow time and widens waveform base. (d) High systemic vascular resistance/afterload: reduced waveform height and narrow base*

Table 6.3 *Possible treatment regimens using PA catheter measurements*

Systolic blood pressure (mmHg)	LV filling pressure (mmHg)	Cardiac index (l/min/m²)	Description	Therapy
<100	<10	<2.5	Hypovolaemia	Volume
<100	10–20	>2.5	Peripheral vasodilation (sepsis)	Pressors
100–150	>20	>2.5	Pulmonary congestion	Diuretics, nitrates
<100	>20	<2.5	LV failure	Vasodilators
<80	>20	<2.0	Cardiogenic shock	Inotropes, vasodilators, balloon pump

Noradrenaline has a specific use in septic shock as a vasopressor: it is used to increase and maintain SVR within the normal range.

Vasodilators such as sodium nitroprusside or nitrates are of use when pulmonary oedema occurs in heart failure, although these drugs can produce a reflex tachycardia if the blood pressure falls. Occasionally, both inotropes and vasodilators are used in combination (*eg* adrenaline and nitroglycerin in severe LVF).

Inotropes and vasodilators can be used safely only where a full range of monitoring is available. They should never be used on ordinary surgical wards and NEVER in the presence of hypovolaemia. Their dose ranges, modes of delivery, etc, are outside the scope of this course; your task is to recognise the clinical conditions that mandate their use and to refer the patient to the appropriate level of care.

SUMMARY

- Adequate cardiovascular function is a prerequisite for survival.
- To determine cardiovascular function accurately and to control manipulative therapy, invasive monitoring is necessary.
- All techniques have complications.
- The monitoring utilised should be appropriate to the specific case in question.

Sepsis and multiple organ failure 7

Objectives

This chapter will help you to:

- Understand the clinical pathophysiology of the septic process.
- Appreciate that prevention, early diagnosis and prompt treatment of sepsis are many times more successful than treatment of established septic shock.

- Understand a system for the management of the septic patient.
- Understand the roles of antibiotics, surgery and other interventions in the management of sepsis.

INTRODUCTION

The number of patients at risk of major sepsis increases progressively each year. Patients such as those with in-dwelling catheters, with prosthetic heart valves, receiving chemotherapy or steroids, with organ transplants, and in intensive care are at particular risk, although in practice many patients with these risk factors have common primary pathologies or operations. Moreover, the progressive ageing of the population and the ability to treat patients with major chronic illness further increases the complexity of management of patients with sepsis. In the USA, septic shock is estimated to account for about 100,000 deaths annually, and the mortality has changed little in the past 20 years. The mortality of surgical patients with major sepsis/septic shock continues at the level of about 50%.

It is important to recognise that the manifestations of infection are brought about by the **release of endogenous mediators**. Such mediator release may result from the presence of bacteria, or from the toxins associated with bacteria, such as endotoxins. Thus, a patient may be severely septic, but with negative blood cultures. The mediators involved in promulgation of the septic response include an array of vasoactive agents, such as nitric oxide, bradykinin, histamine and prosta-

glandins. In combination with a variety of cytokines, they produce a state of **vasodilation**, enhanced **capillary leak** and subsequently **myocardial depression**. Key cytokines involved in the production of the septic response include interleukin-1, tumour necrosis factor (TNF) and interleukin-6, but there are both pro-inflammatory and anti-inflammatory mediators produced. Among other features, these contribute to the patient's pyrexia and hypermetabolism. It is important to recognise that the patient's activated white cells are also a vital component of the systemic manifestation of sepsis. Some production of mediators is needed to combat infection, but an **excessive** or prolonged activation of such cellular/humoral mediator pathways is thought to contribute to the development of multiple organ failure (MOF) in patients with major sepsis. Thus, there is a balance between excessive and inadequate responses to infection. Interindividual variation in the pattern of mediator release and of end-organ responsiveness may play a significant role in determining the initial physiological response to major sepsis, and this in turn may be a key determinant of outcome. Other key determinants of outcome are the initial severity of infection, the timeliness and adequacy of attempts at treatment of the underlying condition, and the patient's general health and consequent ability to withstand the process.

DEFINITIONS OF SEPSIS

There are no clear definitions that permit unfailing identification of the patient with sepsis. Patients fall in a spectrum ranging from the individual with a localised infection (*eg* wound or perianal infection) to those with bacteraemia associated with shock and ensuing organ failure. Four conditions are described that mirror the clinical pictures often seen in sepsis (see box below). All involve a systemic derangement that distinguishes them from localised infection.

DEFINITIONS IN SEPSIS

Systemic inflammatory response syndrome (SIRS) – two of:
- pyrexia (>38°C) or hypothermia (<36°C)
- tachycardia (>90 bpm in absence of beta-blocker)
- tachypnoea (>20/min or a requirement for mechanical ventilation)
- white cell count >12 or <4

Sepsis = SIRS + documented source of infection.

Severe sepsis (confirmed infection) or *sepsis syndrome* (no confirmed infection): SIRS + altered organ perfusion or evidence of dysfunction of one or more organs. Almost any organ or system can be involved, eg:
- CVS: lactate >1.2 mmol/l or SVR <800 dyne/s/cm³
- respiratory: PaO_2/FiO_2 <30 or PaO_2 <9.3 kPa
- renal: urine output <120 ml over four hours
- CNS: Glasgow coma scale (GCS) <15 in absence of sedation/neurological lesion

It is important to note that the identification of organ dysfunction is often initially a **clinical** diagnosis. You should think about organ dysfunction/failure in any critically ill surgical patient who looks breathless and has poor perfusion, confusion, poor urine output or abnormal coagulation.

Septic shock: refractory hypotension in addition to the above, in the presence of invasive infection.

The least severe derangement is SIRS. Many surgical patients will show this and the great majority will recover, but its presence, particularly when it is persistent or if there is tachypnoea, serves as a warning of the **potential** for further deterioration in the absence of prompt treatment. SIRS may result from an infective process or from a severe inflammatory disorder such as pancreatitis, ischaemia, multiple trauma or haemorrhagic shock. When such a response is due to an identified infectious process, this is known as **sepsis**.

The next stage is when organ dysfunction, hypoperfusion or hypotension occurs. This is known as **severe sepsis** (when there is a confirmed infective cause) or **sepsis syndrome** (when there is not). Obviously, the severity of illness increases stepwise and, accordingly, the prognosis worsens.

The septic picture can be caused by surgical and non-surgical factors and, as indicated above, can occur with confirmed infection or in its absence. Although specific criteria for organ dysfunction exist, you should be **actively** looking for clinical evidence of organ derangement (dyspnoea, hypoxia, oliguria, jaundice, thrombocytopenia, etc) in all your susceptible patients.

The essential points of management of the patient with sepsis include:

- early recognition;
- immediate resuscitation;
- localisation of sepsis;
- early and appropriate administration of antibiotics;
- appropriate management of the primary source of sepsis, including the use of surgical or radiological drainage; and
- ongoing reassessment to ensure that the patient continues to improve.

Failure to accomplish any of these promptly will markedly worsen the prognosis.

Table 7.1 shows some causes that you may encounter. The classification might help you to remember them, but a number of the causes could appear in different boxes depending on the stage (*eg* ischaemic gut). Surgical causes often require a surgical solution, but all causes may occur in surgical patients.

Case history 7.1

You are the surgical registrar on the HDU 8am ward round reviewing your patient, a 73-year-old woman with mild chronic obstructive airways disease who had a left hemicolectomy for sigmoid colon cancer (no stoma) six days ago. The house officer tells you that the white cell count was 16.3 yesterday, whereas it was 8.5 the day before.

What would you do?

Assess systematically. ABCs are OK. The only features of note on the charts are a trend to increased heart rate (was 70/min, now 95/min), a temporary pyrexia of 38 °C in the night and some fall-off in urine output (was 50 ml/h, only 25 ml/h for the past three hours but intravenous infusion has been

Table 7.1 *Some causes of the septic process*

	Infective	Non-infective
Non-surgical	Pulmonary	Acute pancreatitis
	Urinary and catheter-related	Reperfusion injury
	Intravenous lines, especially CVP	
	Soft tissue infection	
Surgical	Anastomotic leak	Ischaemic gut
	Biliary, especially if obstructed	Ruptured aorta
	Urinary with obstruction	Major haemorrhage
	Collection/abscess	Trauma
	Infected prosthesis (hip, aortic graft, heart valve, neurosurgical shunt)	
	Necrotic tissue	

behind time). The patient has no specific complaints but has been generally slow to recover. The CVP line is still in, as are the epidural and the urinary catheter. The chest is unchanged – a few basal crackles but stable gas exchange and able to expectorate adequately and without pain. The abdomen is slightly distended; flatus but no faeces has been passed. There is no DVT. The urine is clear.

What now?

Decide and plan! The patient is not quite right but she has no definite signs. There are a number of sources of sepsis (chest, CVP line, urine, urinary catheter, abdomen, wounds, anastomosis). Line, peripheral blood, urine and sputum cultures should be sent. A CXR could be ordered if there is not a recent one. A fluid challenge is started and the physiotherapist is called.

The operation carried out, the anastomosis, the stage of recovery and the fact that the gut has not started working again yet should make you consider an anastomotic leak. You discuss the case with your consultant and arrange a water-soluble rectal contrast study. This shows a small, localised leak, and the consultant thinks that the patient may yet settle. Antibiotics are prescribed and the patient is fasted.

On review

Overall, the patient appears to remain unchanged throughout the next 24 hours. There is one further flicker of pyrexia (37.8 °C). The heart rate remains at 95–100/min. The next morning, the abdomen is still distended and the gut has not worked. The urea has climbed to 10.4 and the patient had a run of fast AF at 5am despite a CVP of +9 and normal

saturations. A 12-lead ECG and cardiac enzymes were normal, but the magnesium level was low; this has been corrected.

Your consultant joins you and together you decide that the failure to respond (abdomen, heart rate) and the recent cardiac and renal effects are more than enough to require surgery to deal with the leak. The patient is optimised and transferred to theatre, where the anastomosis is taken down and the ends exteriorised. The patient returns to HDU and makes an uncomplicated further recovery.

Learning points

- Revise the range of causes of postoperative pyrexia and of sepsis in surgical patients (not the same).
- Anastomotic leaks are not uncommon and can present with an almost infinite variety of features, often between days four and eight. These range from the catastrophic collapse into multiple organ failure to very subtle derangements of vital signs or biochemical parameters. Patients may simply 'fail to progress' as they normally would after that type of operation. Be suspicious about any abnormal or unusual features in patients with anastomoses at this stage. Gut function is usually (but not always) delayed or absent. Often, surgical or radiological intervention is needed, and certainly when the patient has a sizeable leak and/or obvious signs or when a less severe case fails to settle promptly. When there is organ dysfunction, there is a need for prompt action. The type of intervention depends on the site and the previous operation, but leaking small bowel and colonic anastomoses are usually best exteriorised as stomas.

PATIENT ASSESSMENT AND MANAGEMENT

Immediate care

Remember the ABCs. The patient with major sepsis may have a tachypnoea and cardiovascular changes, including a tachycardia and hypotension. Peripheral perfusion may be increased or diminished. The presence of these changes demands at least the administration of high-flow oxygen via a facemask and establishment of intravenous access with volume expansion by appropriate fluid bolus.

Full patient assessment

CHART REVIEW

Vital signs should be reviewed carefully. A tachypnoea, tachycardia, and hypo- or hyperthermia are all consistent with major sepsis. A central venous pressure of 5–10 cmH$_2$O and a urine output greater than 30 ml/h are reasonable guides to the adequacy of initial fluid resuscitation. If hypotension/inadequate perfusion persists despite adequate fluid replacement and CVP monitoring, then inotropic support should be used. In these circumstances, moving the patient to an ICU to allow invasive haemodynamic monitoring (pulmonary artery catheter) should be considered.

HISTORY AND SYSTEMATIC EXAMINATION

Swift assessment of the patient's presenting problem to establish the likely source of sepsis is important. Signs are by no means constant, but positive findings **require action** and certain pointers exist:

- Breathlessness and a productive cough may point to a pulmonary source.
- Abdominal pain or bowel symptoms may point to an abdominal source. An abdominal or pelvic abscess may cause an irritative diarrhoea or an ileus. Anastomotic leaks are common and can be subtle.
- Frequency, dysuria or haematuria might point to the urinary system. Recent catheterisation or instrumentation is a frequent accompaniment to major sepsis associated with the urinary tract.

Beware the combination of obstruction with infection (usually due to a stone), as sepsis may be severe or renal damage may occur rapidly.
- Headache and neck stiffness may point to a source in the CNS. Confusion is, however, a frequent feature of major sepsis and does not necessarily indicate a source in the CNS.

The systemic review should pay particular attention to evaluate chronic health problems and current medication. These may have bearings in terms of a predisposition to sepsis (*eg* use of oral steroids) or may indicate the need for more intensive monitoring (*eg* recent MI). The examination may reveal the patient's peripheries to be warm and pink with a bounding pulse (indicative of mediator-induced vasodilation with a compensatory increase in cardiac output) or, as sepsis progresses with hypovolaemia and myocardial decompensation, the patient may demonstrate pallor, sweating, a thready pulse and cold peripheries. The chest should be examined to exclude atelectasis, an effusion or pneumonia. The abdomen should be checked for localised tenderness, peritonism or ileus. If pelvic sepsis is suspected, a rectal examination is mandatory.

In obtaining the history of events from the patient, notes and other sources, you should be alert to risk factors for the source and severity of sepsis. Think what complications are likely to follow from previous events, particularly recent operations. Common things are common: chest infection, anastomotic leak and central line infection are frequent sources. Timing helps: the chest is a common early cause of postoperative fever or sepsis (from day one onwards); anastomotic leak most commonly occurs between days four and ten and often normal gut function will not have returned; central line infection becomes more frequent in lines more than five to seven days old.

AVAILABLE RESULTS

Review the available results and arrange new investigations.

The white blood cell count may be abnormally high ($> 10 \times 10^9$/l) or low ($< 2 \times 10^9$/l) in major sepsis.

If disseminated intravascular coagulation develops, the platelet count may be low and fibrin degradation products will be elevated. Thrombocytopenia and lesser coagulopathies are common and can be corrected before surgery. A coagulation screen should be checked, particularly if surgery is contemplated.

The urea and electrolytes should be reviewed, with particular attention being paid to renal function. Acute renal failure is a frequent complication of severe sepsis and is preventable in the early stages by adequate volume loading.

Liver function tests (LFTs) may be abnormal if the biliary tree is the primary source of sepsis or bilirubinuria may be detected by urine dipstix. Alternatively, with the development of organ failure, abnormal LFTs may reflect liver dysfunction/failure and a progressively rising bilirubin (eg >300 μmol/l) indicates a poor prognosis.

An ECG should be checked for evidence of ischaemia or arrhythmia. Arterial blood gases should be taken and may show hypoxaemia, with or without a metabolic acidosis.

Aerobic and anaerobic blood cultures are obligatory but will generally be positive in about only 20% of cases. A higher positive culture rate will usually be achieved if the primary source of sepsis can be cultured (pus from an abscess, urine from an infected system, etc). Thus, sputum, urine, drain fluid and pus from wounds should be sent for culture and sensitivity. If the patient is seriously ill, an immediate Gram stain of such specimens can aid appropriate antibiotic prescription. Drawback cultures should be taken from central lines. Consider fungal infection and send fungal cultures if the diagnosis is proving elusive or if there have been multiple previous courses of antibiotics. Usually, 'best-guess' antibiotics will be started, but the value of early cultures will be clear if the response to the first guess is inadequate: by this time, your culture results will be available to guide you, and you should discuss these with the microbiologist if in any doubt.

Case history 7.2

A 61-year-old previously fit woman was admitted to the ward four days ago with acute sigmoid diverticulitis. Initial signs were modest and treatment was started with a second-generation cephalosporin and metronidazole. Fever and leucocytosis settled within 48 hours. Now the patient has suddenly become unwell, with recurrent tenderness in the left iliac fossa, pyrexia of 39.2 °C, tachycardia and hypotension.

What would you do at this stage?

What is your differential diagnosis?

It is clear that the patient has deteriorated markedly despite reasonable treatment for her presumed diagnosis and that a change of treatment is needed. Following resuscitation (including blood cultures and biochemical work-up) and after discussion with her consultant, an experienced surgical trainee takes the patient to theatre for an emergency sigmoid colectomy. A 7-cm pelvic abscess beside the inflamed sigmoid colon is drained and a sample of pus sent for urgent microbiological examination and culture. A Hartmann's procedure (sigmoid colectomy with colostomy and closure of the rectal stump) is carried out, and the patient is returned to the HDU in stable condition. Peroperative antibiotics were given as previously and prescribed for a further five days.

Learning points

- *Anticipate:* from the initial diagnosis and your knowledge of common complications.
- *Resuscitate adequately:* monitor and get help as necessary.
- *Cultures:* blood and source.
- *Antibiotics:* best guess, then selective and in short courses.
- Definitive surgical treatment is essential.

Urine infection is common and can be asymptomatic.

A CXR should be obtained. Further evaluation of possible sites of sepsis include the use of ultrasound, computed tomography (CT) and laparotomy. Remember the adage, pus somewhere, pus nowhere, pus under the diaphragm. Patients who are immunocompromised (eg transplant recipients) may develop opportunistic infections that may require very specific investigation, eg bronchoalveolar lavage or transbronchial biopsy for those with pneumonia.

Daily management plan (if stable)

If the patient is stable, formulate a daily management plan. A list of clear, positive decisions enumerated in the case notes provides a plan for genuine progress. This is the process you undertake on your business ward rounds. The aim is to ensure progress through attention to detail. This gives the patient the best chance of avoiding further deterioration.

- *Fluids:* it is important to maintain the patient on sufficient fluids to allow good tissue perfusion. Remember the importance of uncorrected tissue hypoxia in activating the cytokine cascades. Generally, crystalloids are sufficient. The use of albumin solutions and other colloids when there is severe capillary leak and marked hypoalbuminaemia is highly controversial. Colloids may remain in the circulation longer, but when they escape to the tissues they may worsen oedema. Patients with sepsis syndrome may require up to 10–12 l of fluid in the first 24 hours of resuscitation. Care should be taken to avoid fluid overload.

- *Oxygen:* the main reason for the existence of the cardiovascular system is to deliver oxygen to the tissues and it is essential that the patient does not become hypoxaemic. If this is the case, oxygen should be administered by high-flow oxygen mask; if the patient remains hypoxaemic, then consideration should be given to artificial ventilation. In patients with sepsis, pulmonary function can be confounded by nosocomial infection. The use of enteral nutrition and selective decontamination of the digestive tract may help to prevent the development of the latter.

- *Nutrition:* it is essential to ensure adequate metabolic and nutritional support of the patient in order to optimise the patient's endogenous immune function, thus attention should be paid to the provision of enteral nutrition or, if this is not possible, parenteral nutrition. In the critically ill, however, it is important to recognise the possibility of substrate overload and seldom should patients receive more than 2,000–2,500 kcal/day or 14–18 g/day of nitrogen.

- *Antibiotics:* should be given to the patient as soon as possible and are generally prescribed on a best-guess basis given the clinical scenario. It is sensible to choose an antibiotic that is different from any used recently. A course of treatment should generally be limited to five to seven days and should be in line with local policy. It is important not to forget to **review** the microbiology after 48 hours when cultures are available to ensure that the bacteria causing the infection are sensitive to the prescribed antibiotic. Have a low threshold for discussing cases with the microbiologist. It has been shown clearly that the mortality of patients is significantly lower when appropriate antibiotics are prescribed early in the course of the illness. It is also important to appreciate that **fungi** and atypical organisms can contribute to the sepsis syndrome and to take cultures and prescribe appropriately. Prolonged 'prophylaxis' is detrimental, as superinfection by fungi and antibiotic-resistant *Pseudomonas*, enterococci and staphylococci is encouraged. These infections can carry a high mortality and are difficult to treat. Finally, remember that enteric streptococci account for 10–20% of severe infections related to the abdomen and that they are not sensitive to all common prophylactic antibiotics.

The daily management plan should also include instructions for physiotherapy, particularly with reference to the chest. Patients should receive adequate DVT prophylaxis. In patients with ongoing abdominal sepsis, it is important to have a strategy for drain management. Drains should, in general, be removed as soon as possible since they contravene the integrity of the skin. When a drain is vital (*eg* for control of a fistula), it should be secured carefully (*eg* by suturing).

Diagnosing the cause of deterioration (if unstable)

In a patient with new or ongoing abdominal, pulmonary or soft tissue sepsis, deterioration may be marked by an undulating pyrexia, increasing white cell count, progressive tachycardia, the development of disseminated intravascular coagulation, a metabolic acidosis and multiple organ failure. Alternatively, the patient may simply fail to progress. The presence of such a pattern demands careful clinical review of symptoms and signs, repeat microbiology, review of antibiotic sensitivity and further radiological evaluation with either percutaneous or operative drainage of localised sepsis. **Failure** to diagnose significant sepsis will prove fatal.

Definitive treatment

Definitive treatment is the single most important factor in securing survival. It goes without saying that localised collections of pus generally need either operative or percutaneous drainage and that dead tissue should be excised.

- Severe pulmonary sepsis requires adequate antibiotics and chest physiotherapy and may also require repeat bronchoscopy and toilet of the bronchial tree. This may or may not have to be undertaken with the patient on artificial ventilation.
- In spreading soft tissue infection, it is important to establish adequate drainage and vital to excise necrotic or devitalised tissue as well as giving antibiotics. Repeated examination under anaesthesia with further debridement is usually needed.
- Abdominal sepsis, if localised, may be treated initially with antibiotics or percutaneous drainage, but generally the primary source of sepsis must be removed. Copious intraoperative peritoneal lavage is important, and you should be alert to the development of recurrent sepsis during subsequent assessments of the patient.
- A planned second-look laparotomy may occasionally be useful, especially in patients with equivocal bowel perfusion during the previous procedure.
- In addition to supportive and antibiotic treatment, obstruction to the biliary or urinary system must be relieved (from above or below), usually by endoscopic or radiological means.
- Major sepsis associated with an infected prosthesis most frequently demands removal of the latter (intravenous line, urinary catheter, aortic valve, aortic graft, hip replacement). Sometimes, this is not feasible and careful joint decisions are needed. More commonly, it is important to remain vigilant about the possibility of catheter-associated sepsis, particularly in patients in the HDU or ICU.

Remember that methicillin-resistant *Staphylococcus aureus* (MRSA) is becoming more common in surgical patients. It is important to distinguish between patients who are colonised carriers and those with MRSA sepsis. However, while MRSA colonisation does not present major problems in most patients, it does in those patients with prostheses (aortic valves, aortic grafts, hip replacements), where it is associated with a very high mortality. Often, the only treatment is removal of the prosthesis and long-term antibiotics. Microbiological help is essential.

Prevent – diagnose – act!

Case history 7.3

When on call, you are asked to review the patient discussed in Case history 7.2 72 hours following surgery. She had improved for 48 hours and was returned to the ward, but she is now breathless and pyrexial again (38.3°C), having been apyrexial since four hours after surgery. Her blood pressure is normal, but she is tachycardic (115/min), tachypnoeic (28/min) and poorly perfused. Urine output has fallen off over the last four hours to 12 ml in the last hour. The chest seems clear. Her abdomen is distended and quiet. The stoma has not worked properly yet. The pelvic drain has produced 40 ml serous fluid today only. You give high-flow oxygen (12 l/min) and start a fluid challenge of 500 ml 0.9% saline stat.

The house officer had checked bloods and a CXR. Apart from a leucocytosis (17.1), results are unremarkable. There are no diagnostic features on the CXR. There are no signs of DVT, and prescribed DVT prophylaxis (subcutaneous heparin and thromboembolic deterrent (TED) stockings) are in place. You perform a cautious rectal examination but find no obvious abnormality. Blood gases are now checked and show the following: PaO_2 (on FiO_2 of 0.6) 11.4 kPa, pH 7.29 and base excess − 7.2.

You move the patient to HDU. When the results come back, you decide that the patient has been acidotic and hypoxic and that you have barely corrected the hypoxia with the facemask oxygen. After 1000 ml of saline, there is a little improvement in perfusion but no change in the heart rate, and urine output is only 15 ml in the hour since you were called.

What would you do now?

What is your differential diagnosis?

The patient remains breathless and you have neither a diagnosis nor any further intervention of obvious help at your disposal. You request an urgent review by the ICU. As the patient still seems underperfused, you give a further fluid challenge, while the house officer checks the ECG (normal).

The ICU team arrives and assesses the patient. They share your concern and think that ventilation will be needed; transfer is arranged. You inform your consultant, who asks to be kept informed. During transfer, the patient becomes more breathless and is intubated shortly after arriving in the ICU. The positive-pressure ventilation reduces cardiac filling; despite further fluid loading, inotropes are required to support the cardiovascular system. Urine output tails off. A pulmonary artery catheter is inserted. The CXR taken to check the position of the catheter also shows some diffuse bilateral shadowing, suggestive of ARDS. You update your consultant, who comes to examine the patient. No cause for deterioration has yet been found.

Given the previous operation and the leucocytosis, recurrent abdominal sepsis is suspected. The patient is too unstable for CT, so repeat laparotomy is arranged and carried out by the consultant. The bowel is intact but two abscesses are found between loops of small intestine and a left subphrenic abscess is identified; these are drained and lavaged. More pus is sent for culture.

The patient returns to the ICU for full cardiac, respiratory and renal support. The culture result from the pus taken at the first operation has grown a coliform resistant to prescribed antibiotics but sensitive to netilmicin. Treatment is changed accordingly and a seven-day course started. The patient slowly begins to improve over the succeeding 72 hours.

Learning points

- Sepsis can progress rapidly: an escalating degree of support, often out of working hours, may be required. Your role is to recognise and treat the many patients with 'minor' sepsis who respond adequately on the ward, but also to recognise the patient who is not responding and who needs ICU help.
- A diagnosis that accounts adequately for any septic deterioration is essential: this allows for definitive treatment.
- Early cultures can help target later treatment: the right antibiotic is important.

MANAGEMENT OF MULTIPLE ORGAN FAILURE

Due to the severity of the initial insult or when there is a persistence of an activated systemic inflammatory response, a patient may develop dysfunction or failure of one or more organ systems (cardiovascular, pulmonary, renal, gut, liver, haematological, CNS). When three or more systems have failed, the ensuing mortality approaches 80–100% and, once one organ system has failed, others typically follow, like a collapsing pack of cards. It is important to appreciate this phenomenon of organ failure amplification and to strive to support as far

as possible each organ system to avoid each further adverse event (eg ventilation, haemofiltration/ haemodialysis, inotropic support, nutritional support, use of blood products).

Respiratory failure can result from lung infection (often superadded to pre-existing chronic airway disease) or from ARDS. ARDS is a diffuse inflammatory process of both lungs. Like SIRS, it is seen most commonly in sepsis but also after pancreatitis or trauma. The lungs become waterlogged due to extravasation of inflammatory fluid and cells. It quickly becomes very difficult to ventilate the patient. On the ward, patients develop ARDS over a few hours. Pulmonary signs are often minimal or non-specific, the patient simply being breathless, progressively tachypnoeic, hypoxic and then cyanotic. A CXR will show bilateral infiltrates but this may lag behind the clinical picture. Ventilation is almost always needed, and expert ICU help should be obtained at an early stage; *suspicion* is the key to diagnosis. If the patient is already ventilated, then ventilatory pressures and necessary FiO_2 increase as ARDS progresses (see Chapter 3).

Cardiovascular failure in MOF due to sepsis typically results from three main factors: marked loss of peripheral vascular tone, continuing loss of circulating volume due to leaky capillaries, and myocardial depression. Arrhythmias can exert a further effect. Close monitoring of preload, cardiac function and afterload is usual. Fluid loading, the initial step, is occasionally sufficient on its own, but inotropic support is often needed. Preference varies according to local policies, but many intensivists would use noradrenaline to increase peripheral vascular tone, often in conjunction with other agents to increase cardiac contractility.

Renal failure is common in MOF and often is established during the early stages before hypovolaemia is corrected. Circulating nephrotoxins (see Chapter 8) compound this. Renal function will return when perfusion and oxygenation are adequate, but until this occurs renal replacement therapy is needed.

Failure of other systems (gut, brain, clotting system, etc) occurs again, due partly to the direct effects of the pathology or surgery and partly to systemic inflammation and hypoxia. The poor prognosis of MOF has been indicated above, but for there to be **any** real prospect of recovery the underlying cause or source of sepsis must be dealt with.

Nosocomial (hospital-acquired) infection is common in patients treated in ICUs and compounds the MOF process. The source of infection is often endogenous. However, the decision to give antibiotics for a positive culture (*eg* of *Pseudomonas*) should be balanced carefully by the presence of a host response to such bacteria, the site of the potential infection, and the need to avoid superinfection or antibiotic resistance. Discuss the issues with your microbiologist. It is often the case that patients with MOF die with concurrent infection rather than because of such infection, probably due to immunological failure.

The recognition of the role of endogenous mediators in sepsis syndrome and the advent of biotechnology resulted in several large multicentre randomised trials using monoclonal antibodies or antagonists to various sepsis mediators, including endotoxin, TNF and interleukin-1. These trials have generally not reduced mortality, although there are one or two areas of promise (*eg* protein C therapy). It is now recognised that the redundancy in the inflammatory response is such that, if one component is removed, another mediator will continue the response. Moreover, if the pool of endogenous antagonists (*eg* interleukin-1 receptor antagonist or soluble TNF receptors) is replete, then addition of exogenous antagonists is unlikely to be efficacious. It remains clear that these treatments are unlikely to **ever** replace the established basic principles of management, although time will tell whether a substantial adjuvant role can be identified.

Case history 7.4

The patient seen in Case histories 7.2 and 7.3 deteriorates again overnight, needing increased vasoconstrictors, inotropes and oxygen, highly suggestive of sepsis. A full infection screen of cultures has been taken by the time you arrive, and the central lines have been changed over guidewires by the ICU staff. There are no clinical features to suggest recurrent intra-abdominal sepsis. A CT scan is arranged and is negative. The patient has had several recent courses of antibiotics and there is no clear best-guess antibiotic to use that has not been tried already.

What is your differential diagnosis?
Six hours later, the patient is no better and a joint discussion is held among surgeons, ICU staff and the microbiologist. No cultures are available, but fungi were seen on samples from the urinary catheter and one of the removed central lines. It is decided to commence amphotericin and fluconazole for presumed fungal sepsis.

After a four-week course and several other complications, the patient is discharged to the ward.

Learning points
- Surgical patients on the ICU with sepsis and MOF run a roller-coaster course, often with a range of complications, some surgical and some medical. An active surgical input to care helps manage these effectively.
- Multiple courses of antibiotics, gastrointestinal perforation, critical illness and multiple monitoring lines are all risk factors for fungal sepsis; many of these factors pertain in a majority of surgical patients.
- Fungal sepsis may present with obscure signs — a failure to progress. Identification of fungi within the blood, abdomen or urine (or at any two other sites) would prompt many intensivists to discuss antifungal therapy with their microbiologist and surgeon.

Established septic shock or MOF is thus really only treatable by *prevention* through attention to detail:

- *Preoperatively*, the general health of the patient should be optimised (coexisting diseases, nutrition) and foci of sepsis dealt with.
- *Perioperatively*, prophylactic antibiotics should be given and surgery executed in a rapid, clean and haemostatic manner in order to prevent complications. Operate electively when possible and avoid hypothermia.
- *Postoperatively*, assess clinically and monitor closely to detect problems at an early stage and deal with these quickly and comprehensively. Be alert to 'occult' hypoxia and hypovolaemia. Use prophylactic measures such as chest physiotherapy and resume oral intake/enteral feeding at the earliest opportunity. Likewise, remove lines and tubes and employ short courses of targeted antibiotics. In the event of a septic complication, adequate resuscitation and early definitive treatment should reduce the chance of full-blown sepsis developing.

SUMMARY

- Sepsis is a mediator disease.
- Prevention is best.
- Clinical signs may be obvious or covert.
- Treatment is much easier at an early stage.
- The principles of management are:
  - rapid resuscitation to restore oxygenation and perfusion;
  - continued optimal organ support;
  - diagnosis and eradication of the source of sepsis and any pus;
  - judicious and appropriate antibiotic treatment after cultures; and
  - reassessment to ensure continued progress.

Objectives

This chapter will help you to:

- Understand the functions of the kidney.
- Be familiar with the five rules of renal failure.
- Be able to discuss the causes of renal failure in the surgical patient.

- Be able to discuss the prevention and management of renal failure in the critically ill surgical patient.

INTRODUCTION

Abnormal renal function is common in the critically ill surgical patient. Oliguria is one of the most common reasons for a doctor being called to see a patient following surgery, and acute renal failure requiring renal replacement therapy (RRT) is seen in up to 10% of surgical patients requiring unplanned intensive care. Acute renal failure is often preventable in the surgical patient, in many cases by adequate fluid therapy alone.

FUNCTIONS OF THE KIDNEYS

The primary functions of the kidneys are:

- fluid, electrolyte and hydrogen ion homeostasis;
- excretion of water-soluble waste products of metabolism (eg urea);
- excretion of water-soluble drugs; and
- endocrine functions, eg renin–angiotensin, erythropoietin, vitamin D.

ACUTE AND CHRONIC RENAL FAILURE

Definitions

Chronic renal failure (CRF) is defined as the chronic irreversible loss of nephrons, resulting in permanent impairment of solute excretion.

Acute renal failure is defined as the sudden (and often recoverable) impairment of the kidneys' ability to excrete the nitrogenous waste products of metabolism.

The important difference between these two conditions is that CRF is usually caused by a variety of chronic medical conditions (eg longstanding diabetes mellitus and hypertension) whereas acute renal failure is often seen in surgical patients and is caused by loss of renal perfusion as a result of shock, sepsis or nephrotoxins.

PHYSIOLOGICAL BASIS OF RENAL FUNCTION

The kidneys filter 125 ml/min of plasma water through a semipermeable basement membrane that restricts the passage of solute on the basis of molecular size and charge. This restriction prevents the passage of albumin and solute greater than 68,000 Da. This filtrate enters the renal tubular system, where the vast majority of the filtered solute and water essential to maintain normal body function is reabsorbed in its proximal section. Fine control of sodium, potassium, hydrogen ions and water is effected in the distal tubule. A small quantity of solute is secreted directly into the tubules.

The energy necessary to generate glomerular filtration is produced by the action of the heart and circulation in maintaining an adequate perfusion pressure. Reduction in renal perfusion from whatever cause immediately stresses the kidney and leads to increased proximal tubular reabsorption of sodium and water from the normal 55% towards 100%. A minimal volume of filtrate reaches the distal nephron, which immediately impairs the kidneys' ability to excrete potassium, hydrogen ion and water.

> Without adequate perfusion, the kidneys cannot function.

The energy required for tubular function is derived from oxidative metabolism in the mitochondria of the proximal and distal tubular cells. The tubular cells deep in the medulla of the kidney operate at the limit of oxidative cellular metabolism and are very sensitive to ischaemia or hypoxia. The cells of the thick ascending limb of the loop of Henle are the most vulnerable. Furthermore, the underperfused kidney is much more sensitive to other insults, *eg* sepsis and nephrotoxins.

The five rules of renal failure

1 The kidneys cannot function without adequate perfusion.
2 Renal perfusion is dependent on adequate blood pressure.
3 A surgical patient with poor urine output usually requires more fluid.
4 Absolute anuria is usually due to urinary tract obstruction.
5 Poor urine output in a surgical patient is not due to furosemide (frusemide) deficiency.

Case history 8.1

Eight hours following an elective abdominal aortic aneurysm replacement, a 68-year-old man develops oliguria despite receiving 100 ml of 0.9% saline per hour and with no major change in pulse rate or blood pressure. There have been no obvious signs of haemorrhage or excess loss from the nasogastric tube. The CVP is 10 cmH$_2$O, but the HDU nurse feels that the trace is unreliable and 'positional' and suggests that the patient is suboptimally perfused. Haemoglobin is 11.1 g/dl. The SHO recommends a dose of furosemide (80 mg i.v.) to improve the urine output. This improves the urine output to 100 ml for two hours, after which it falls again to 20 ml/h. The

specialist registrar on call prescribes a further dose of furosemide (40 mg i.v.) by telephone. This has no effect, and the ICU consultant is contacted. He resites the CVP line and the measurement is found to be very low. Immediate circulatory volume expansion, however, does not restore urinary output. By the next day, the plasma creatinine and urea have risen rapidly and renal replacement therapy is required. The patient has a long and complicated course and dies of multiple organ failure three weeks later.

Learning points
- Adequate renal perfusion is the critical factor – this is often achieved simply.
- Insensible and tissue fluid losses continue after surgery – postoperative hypovolaemia is common and may not be caused by acute postoperative haemorrhage.
- CVP readings complement clinical assessment and are not a substitute.
- Consider advice from nursing staff.
- Furosemide will not salvage renal function in a hypovolaemic patient.
- The window of opportunity for successful simple treatment is narrow.
- The five rules of renal failure would have helped in the management of this patient.

SIMPLE ASSESSMENT OF RENAL FUNCTION

Urine volume

Urine volume is the simplest measure of renal function and a very common reason for a doctor being called to see a postoperative surgical patient. The body produces a number of solute particles per day, depending on diet, tissue breakdown, therapeutic agents and poisons. There is a minimum volume of urine into which this solute load may be concentrated. This minimum volume depends on both the amount of solute to be excreted and the concentrating ability of the kidney. The latter depends upon age (the very young and the elderly have a limited ability to concentrate solute in their urine) and the presence of acute or chronic renal disease.

In a normal healthy adult, the minimum urine volume is approximately 500 ml/day. This allows for the normal adult daily solute load of around 600 mosmol and a maximum concentrating ability of 1,200 mosmol/kg of water. Therefore, if the daily urine volume is inadequate, there will be accumulation of nitrogenous and other solute waste, with a rise in plasma levels of urea and creatinine. However, even if the urine volume is greater than this minimum value, renal function may still be abnormal. For example, when there is an increased solute load following trauma, major surgery or sepsis, a **much greater volume** of urine will be required to excrete the daily solute load.

> **DEFINITIONS**
> - Normal urine output in adults is usually 1 ml/kg/h (*ie* for a 70-kg man, 70 ml/h).
> - Oliguria is defined as the production of less than 400 ml/day in the adult (< 17 ml/h).
> - Anuria means the absence of urine, but the term is conventionally applied to daily urine production of less than 100 ml/day in the adult.

Plasma urea and creatinine

The blood levels of these waste products of metabolism are normally maintained at a steady state as a result of the combined effects of the rate of production by dietary intake and metabolism, and the rate of excretion by antidiuretic hormone (ADH) release and adequate renal function. Plasma urea concentration falls during starvation and is increased by an acute protein load, such as with gastrointestinal haemorrhage, trauma or major surgery. However, urea is a less reliable measure of acute renal function change than creatinine, which is produced at a more constant rate in relation to lean body mass (except during acute rhabdomyolysis) and is not concentrated within the renal medulla.

MANAGEMENT OF RENAL FAILURE

In surgical patients, four different patient scenarios are often encountered:

1 An elective surgical patient with preoperative chronic renal impairment.
2 Acute renal impairment in a critically ill surgical patient (pre- or postoperative).
3 A surgical patient with established acute renal failure.
4 A surgical patient with CRF.

Preoperative management of renal impairment

It is not uncommon to find abnormalities of a patient's urea and electrolytes preoperatively. In the elective situation, it may be appropriate to postpone surgery and investigate the cause. Common causes of CRF include:

- hypertension,
- diabetes mellitus,
- renal artery stenosis,
- glomerulonephritis,
- diuretic therapy,
- non-steroidal anti-inflammatory drugs (NSAIDs), and
- angiotensin-converting enzyme (ACE) inhibitors.

Appropriate investigations include a renal opinion, testing urine for infection, management of hypertension, renal ultrasound to detect small (chronically damaged) kidneys (usually less than 11 cm length) and a duplex scan for renal artery stenosis. It is also important to stop any potentially **nephrotoxic** drugs such as NSAIDs and ACE inhibitors.

In the emergency situation, it is usually appropriate to proceed to surgery with adequate volume resuscitation, maintenance of cardiac output, avoidance of nephrotoxic drugs and treatment of sepsis. Any persisting renal impairment is then managed postoperatively with a similar approach and renal replacement therapy (RRT) if necessary.

Management of acute renal impairment

The principles of the immediate management of a patient with acute renal impairment include:

- Assess and correct any respiratory or circulatory deficit.
- Manage immediately life-threatening consequences of renal impairment.
- Exclude obstruction of the urinary tract.
- Careful search for the underlying cause and prompt correction.
- Summon help from appropriately trained specialists.

The most obvious indicator of impaired renal function is the development of oliguria or anuria. Absolute anuria (no urine) strongly suggests obstruction of the lower urinary tract, which must be excluded rapidly (usually with an ultrasound scan). Remember to exclude a blocked urinary catheter.

> Complete anuria means lower urinary tract obstruction until proven otherwise.

Acute renal impairment may also be detected by rising serum urea and creatinine levels. In the critically ill surgical patient, there are usually several potential insults that combine to injure the kidney, a frequent combination being hypovolaemia, sepsis and nephrotoxic drugs.

Case history 8.2

A 45-year-old previously healthy woman presents with jaundice and cholangitis. She has pyrexia (38.4 °C) and tachycardia (115/min) but she is normotensive. She is treated with intravenous antibiotics and fluids, and her condition improves. An urgent ultrasound scan suggests stones in the common bile duct. Endoscopic retrograde cholangiopancreatography (ERCP) is booked for later in the week.

The ERCP proves difficult, and adequate drainage of the common bile duct is not achieved. A percutaneous transhepatic cholangiogram (PTC) is scheduled for the following day, but 12 hours after the ERCP the patient becomes hypotensive and pyrexial. The serum amylase and an abdominal X-ray are normal. Treatment is started with oxygen and intravenous fluid challenges, and the intravenous antibiotics are continued. The patient is transferred to the HDU, and a CVP line is inserted (+10 cmH$_2$O). The blood pressure is restored but the urine output remains poor; by the following morning, the urea is 25.7 and creatinine is 229. The patient is not on any nephrotoxic drugs.

It is clear that definitive treatment in the form of biliary drainage is needed urgently. An emergency PTC is arranged for later the same day. The PTC is performed by a consultant radiologist, with an anaesthetist and an HDU nurse in attendance, and with portable monitoring in place. Successful biliary drainage is achieved, but the patient requires several days of haemofiltration on the HDU. She eventually makes a slow but full recovery, and has a successful ERCP subsequently and later elective laparoscopic cholecystectomy.

Learning points
- Multiple factors often contribute to acute renal failure in surgical critical care – biliary obstruction, sepsis and hypovolaemia are a potent combination.
- Patients with obstructive jaundice tend to be dehydrated and need adequate fluid therapy and clinical monitoring. Procedures such as ERCP and PTC can exacerbate hypovolaemia or sepsis in a number of ways, and adequate periprocedural antibiotics and intravenous fluids are needed in such cases – they are easily overlooked.
- Timely definitive treatment of the underlying cause is usually the key to success.

PATIENT HISTORY

An accurate history, ideally from the patient and supplemented by information from relatives, friends, the general practitioner and hospital case notes, is essential. Particular note must be made of any past history or family history of renal disease, hypertension, diabetes mellitus or vascular disease. A comprehensive history of all medications (including contrast media), prescribed or otherwise, is essential.

EXAMINATION

Specific physical signs associated with renal disease apart from examination of the urine are generally few. Occasionally, physical signs may suggest the diagnosis, *eg* skin lesions in vasculitic diseases that may present with intra-abdominal catastrophes or the palpably enlarged kidneys of polycystic disease. Prostatic enlargement or a palpable bladder will strongly suggest urinary tract obstruction. An essential part of the examination rests in testing the urine for the presence of blood or protein. Marked proteinuria or microscopically confirmed haematuria with casts suggests a primary renal insult.

ULTRASOUND

Obstruction of the lower urinary tract (or urinary catheter) must be ruled out immediately in the totally anuric patient and within 24 hours in all other cases of renal impairment. Ultrasound performed by a trained radiologist is the preferred method. Rarely, in the early stages of obstruction, the collecting system will not show dilation. Ultrasound will also give information about renal size (small kidneys suggest chronic disease). Renal artery stenosis may be detected by duplex scan.

RADIOLOGY

Plain abdominal X-ray may be of value to detect renal calculus disease, but ultrasound will generally give more information. CT scanning gives the best anatomical detail and, with the use of contrast, gives information about renal function. Intravenous urography gives similar information, but more and better detail is gained by CT. Remember that all contrast media are potentially nephrotoxic, particularly in patients who are extracellular fluid (ECF) depleted or who have myeloma, CRF or diabetes mellitus. Radionuclide studies can be used to determine renal blood flow, renal function and the presence of obstruction, but formal angiography will be required to identify specific vascular lesions, *eg* renal artery injury or stenosis that may be amenable to treatment.

TREATMENT

Restoration of renal perfusion

In all cases, adequate renal perfusion must be restored and maintained as soon as possible. Given the liability of tubular cells to hypoxic damage, provision of oxygen is important. There are many reasons why surgical patients become hypovolaemic (bleeding, third space loss, fluid redistribution, starvation, increased insensible losses), and in many situations oliguria may be corrected simply by restoring circulating and ECF volume. If there is not a rapid response, then CVP monitoring will be needed. Some patients may also require inotropes (with invasive blood pressure monitoring) to maintain mean arterial blood pressure if oliguria persists once the circulating volume has been shown to be adequate. Refer to Chapter 5 to revise the approach and typical volumes of fluid needed. There is no convincing evidence to show that low-dose ('renal-dose') dopamine, diuretics or mannitol has any place in the prevention or treatment of renal impairment.

Relief of urinary tract obstruction

Drainage of an infected obstructed urinary tract is a medical emergency. This should be achieved promptly by urethral or suprapubic catheterisation for bladder outlet obstruction and by percutaneous nephrostomy or retrograde catheterisation of the ureters for upper urinary tract obstruction. Antibiotic cover is essential but often forgotten.

Removal and avoidance of nephrotoxic agents

A history of administration of nephrotoxic drugs must be sought and their administration stopped if possible. Common examples are aminoglycoside antibiotics (*eg* gentamicin), NSAIDs, ACE inhibitors, opioids and beta-blockers. These drugs impair renal function in a dose-dependent way, and their continuing administration in the face of diminishing renal function will produce a positive-feedback loop, making the problem worse. X-ray contrast media are also nephrotoxic and may be the cause of the renal insufficiency. Any drug excreted predominantly by the kidney must have its dosing interval changed when renal function is reduced to avoid toxic side effects. One example is the severe neurotoxicity caused by imipenem if administered in normal dose to patients with renal impairment.

Treatment of underlying cause

In many surgical situations, the kidney is the passive victim of another process. The acute renal insufficiency will not be corrected adequately by these general measures unless the **primary surgical condition is corrected** promptly after appropriate resuscitation, *eg* resection of ischaemic gut, treatment of sepsis or revascularisation of an ischaemic leg.

Rhabdomyolysis

Rhabdomyolysis is the breakdown of damaged muscle (*eg* following acute limb ischaemia or crush injury) with release of myoglobin into the circulation. This condition is usually diagnosed by knowledge of the appropriate underlying cause, dark brown urine (myoglobinuria), positive urinalysis for myoglobin and acute renal impairment. It may be possible to prevent progression to established severe acute renal failure by aggressive volume expansion plus the administration of sodium bicarbonate to alkalinise the urine. The aim is to produce a diuresis and limit the toxic effect of acid products of myoglobin breakdown on the renal tubular cells. The window of opportunity to prevent this effect is small, and if missed acute renal failure requiring

RRT is the inevitable consequence. Early recognition of the potential problem and rapid remedial action are essential.

Decision to stop fluid loading

If the patient does not respond to fluid loading alone, then you will have moved the patient to the HDU, inserted a CVP line, ensured the circulation is full and perhaps started an inotrope (with appropriate senior advice and assistance). You will also have looked for toxins and underlying surgical problems to correct, as indicated above. However, in a few patients, you will still reach the stage where you are starting to think that the patient is passing into established renal failure. Obviously, you will not wish to overload the patient's circulation and cause pulmonary oedema, and you will slow down the intravenous fluids and seek further help from the renal team and the ICU.

In other patients, you will be unsure from the outset whether the patient has pre-renal or renal failure. Clinical circumstances and the response to judicious fluids will give an indication and will also treat any correctable component. Additionally, urine sodium concentration can help (low in pre-renal failure, higher in established renal failure) but this is seldom of great help in acute surgical practice.

Management of established acute renal failure

RENAL REPLACEMENT THERAPY

If acute renal insufficiency does not respond to the above measures and progresses to established acute renal failure, RRT will be required. This may be by dialysis (peritoneal or haemo) or by haemofiltration, or by a combination of the two. The indications for commencing RRT are:

- uncontrollable hyperkalaemia;
- severe salt and water overload, usually with pulmonary oedema;
- uraemia (to prevent encephalopathy); and
- acidosis.

The first two indications are usually self-evident, but the threshold for treatment of uraemia is more controversial. The rapidity of rise of blood urea as well as the absolute level is taken into account in light of the clinical situation. A rising blood urea

level of more than 35 mmol/l unresponsive to other therapies is an absolute indication for initiating RRT. RRT is discontinued once renal function becomes sufficient to allow adequate clearance of nitrogenous waste products.

DIALYSIS

Dialysis is a process by which small-molecular-weight solute equilibrates between a blood compartment and a dialysate compartment separated by a semipermeable membrane (in the dialysis machine or the peritoneum). Small-molecular-weight solute waste moves across the membrane down a concentration gradient. The dialysate contains normal solute in the appropriate concentration to maintain normal blood concentrations, *eg* sodium, calcium, magnesium, chloride, etc.

HAEMOFILTRATION

In haemofiltration, plasma water is driven under pressure through a semipermeable membrane in a large volume using a process similar to that in the glomerulus. Water and solute are then replaced from a separate source to replace the essential components filtered, and the filtrate is discarded. The clearance of small-molecular-weight solute is higher in haemodialysis, but the clearance of intermediate-molecular-weight solute is greater in haemofiltration. It has been suggested that haemofiltration is less stressful on the circulation in the critically ill patient.

HYPERKALAEMIA

Significant hyperkalaemia or a rapidly rising serum potassium requires **immediate treatment** to prevent life-threatening dysrhythmias and cardiac arrest. Absolute figures are difficult to define, because the rate of rise of serum potassium is more significant. Longstanding hyperkalaemia is less dangerous than a recent rise. A rise to a level greater than 6.0 mmol/l should cause concern and a reason should be found. All iatrogenic causes of hyperkalaemia should be identified and stopped. If levels are higher than 6.0 mmol/l and there are ECG signs of toxicity (peaked T waves and ventricular arrhythmias) following restoration of circulating volume and renal perfusion, then intravenous calcium, followed by glucose with or without insulin, sodium bicarbonate or possibly salbutamol by infusion should be administered immediately, with ECG monitoring (see Table 8.1). No potassium is removed from the body by these therapies; it is moved into the intracellular space.

If these measures are insufficient to control hyperkalaemia or if the patient is excessively fluid overloaded, then dialysis or haemofiltration will be required to remove potassium from the body. The use of ion-exchange resins that bind potassium within the gut should be avoided unless there is no alternative. These are slow to act and are extremely unpleasant for the patient to take and the nursing staff to administer. Given orally, they are also potent constipating agents. They will not control situations when large amounts of potassium are released, *eg* in crush injury, burns and major trauma, situations in which the other conservative measures also tend to fail. All potassium supplements must be stopped, as must all other drugs that reduce normal renal potassium excretion (*eg* potassium-sparing diuretics, ACE inhibitors).

Recovery phase of established acute renal failure

As individual nephrons recover, the kidney behaves as in CRF. Because only a proportion of the nephron mass has recovered, each nephron has a much higher daily solute load to excrete. There is therefore a major limitation in the kidneys' ability to conserve sodium, potassium, bicarbonate and water. With modern management of renal failure, major problems of huge losses of water and electrolyte are unusual. The major exception is in post-obstructive

diuresis, where losses will need to be measured and replaced as appropriate. It is important that the recovering kidney is not exposed to further insults in the form of hypotension or nephrotoxic agents, *eg* NSAIDs, to which it is very sensitive. By six months, the kidney will normally have recovered to 85–90% of its premorbid function, although some patients will not recover renal function and will progress to CRF, requiring permanent RRT or transplantation.

Chronic renal failure

CRF is defined as chronic irreversible loss of nephron mass resulting in permanent impairment of solute waste excretion. These patients are usually under the care of a nephrologist and may or may not require permanent RRT.

Patients with CRF have much less ability to compensate for circulatory stress and to resist the effects of nephrotoxins. A simple example is the patient with significant CRF (creatinine 300 mmol/l) who is fasted overnight before surgery. This will cause mild intravascular volume depletion. As there are far fewer nephrons, each has to carry increased solute; this acts as an osmotic diuretic, which prevents concentration of the urine to a degree dependent upon the severity of the CRF. This prevents maximum sodium and water retention until there has been a significant fall in glomerular filtration rate secondary to a contracted circulating volume. Thus, the patient becomes dehydrated and renal function diminishes further. Depriving patients with CRF of oral fluid for any significant length of time (more than

Table 8.1 *Emergency therapy for hyperkalaemia*

Drug	Mechanism	Effect
Calcium gluconate i.v. 10–30 ml 10% solution	Membrane stabilisation	Rapid effect, short action *Drawback:* short action
Dextrose i.v. 50 ml 50% solution bolus, then infusion of 10% solution plus insulin 10–20 units/100 g of dextrose	Transfer of potassium into cells	Rapid effect, intermediate action *Drawback:* central line preferred
Sodium bicarbonate intravenous infusion 1.26% or 1.4% solution at 100 ml/h. A small volume of 8.4% (1 mmol/ml) solution may be required initially to gain control	Transfer of potassium into cells	Rapid effect, intermediate action, best with metabolic acidosis *Drawback:* beware sodium overload
Salbutamol 5–10 μg/min intravenous infusion	Transfer of potassium into cells	Rapid effect, short action *Drawback:* tachycardia, vasodilator

four to six hours) should be avoided unless fluid is given intravenously.

Many patients with severe CRF will be chronically anaemic. Sudden rapid correction of the anaemia by transfusion will acutely impair renal function by altering the flow characteristics of the blood. Transfusion for chronic anaemia is seldom necessary and should be done slowly.

All patients with renal transplants who develop surgical disease must be managed in conjunction with their nephrologist or transplant centre. Skilled assistance will be required to manage their immunosuppression and reduce the likelihood of an acute rejection episode.

Acute renal failure is not a cause of death unless a decision has been made not to treat the resultant uraemia. The cause of death is the underlying condition.

SUMMARY

- Remember the five rules of renal failure:
  - the kidneys cannot function without adequate perfusion;
  - renal perfusion is dependent on adequate blood pressure;
  - a surgical patient with poor urine output usually requires more fluid;
  - absolute anuria is usually due to urinary tract obstruction; and
  - poor urine output in a surgical patient is not due to furosemide deficiency.
- Resuscitate adequately.
- Avoid nephrotoxins.
- Deal with any underlying cause.

The abdomen in critical surgical illness

Objectives

This chapter will help you to:

- Understand the frequency and rapidity with which abdominal disease, particularly as a septic source, can cause critical illness.
- Be aware of the importance of achieving timely resuscitation, diagnosis and definitive treatment in order to prevent established organ failure.
- Recognise features of an acute abdomen that would indicate the need for HDU/ICU support.

- Recognise the difficulty of diagnosis, particularly in the ICU and after recent surgery.
- Be aware of the commoner complications of surgery that can occur in the critically ill and the methods for their prevention.
- Be knowledgeable in the management of wounds, stomas and drains on the ICU.

INTRODUCTION

Due to the nature of its viscera and the operations performed thereon, the abdomen harbours a remarkable propensity for causing critical illness, mainly through infection, sepsis and haemorrhage. These processes can occur as part of a range of diseases or as complications following almost any intra-abdominal surgery (see Table 9.1). Deterioration can be rapid and obvious, but the diagnosis may be delayed due to hidden or non-specific early features. Once

ICU support is necessary, however, mortality approaches 70%, so the prevention of multiple organ failure through the early detection of deterioration and definitive treatment of the cause is vital. Problems can be anticipated through the approaches already outlined in this book. Early transfer to the HDU or ICU will often be needed. Abdominal problems can recur or develop afresh in patients in the ICU or other critical care areas. Making the diagnosis, while vital to survival, can prove very difficult. Finally, once on the ICU, assessment of the abdomen

Table 9.1 *Common causes of critical abdominal illness*

Infarcted tissue, particularly strangulated bowel or intestinal ischaemia

Intestinal perforation

Acute haemorrhage: ruptured aortic aneurysm or gastrointestinal haemorrhage (particularly recurrent haemorrhage) or associated with multiple trauma

Postoperative bleeding: 'surgical' or in relation to stress gastritis or disseminated intravascular coagulation (DIC)

Biliary infection with obstructive jaundice

Pancreatitis in predicted severe disease (on Ranson or Imrie criteria)

When second-look surgery is anticipated

Intestinal obstruction, with marked intercompartment fluid shifts or pre-renal failure

Prolonged postoperative ileus

Postoperative complications following intestinal leakage

Old age, concomitant medical disease or delayed diagnosis compounding the above or combined with simple pathology to produce actual or threatened organ dysfunction and care of surgical facets of care such as drains, wounds and stomas are areas where all surgeons, including trainees, can offer useful expertise to the ICU team's management of the complex patient with organ failure.

Case history 9.1

A 71-year-old woman presents through the emergency room with a four-hour history of worsening upper abdominal and back pain, nausea and vomiting. Her family doctor referred her, noting only a five-year history of mild hypertension. On examination on arrival, she was shocked and cyanosed but responded well to oxygen and intravenous fluid therapy. A CXR was normal, but an abdominal film showed a sentinel loop of proximal jejunum. An ECG was normal.

What is your diagnosis?
Selected blood results were as follows (conventional units):

Haemoglobin 16.1
White cell count 24.2
Amylase 8900
Sodium 141
Potassium 3.2
Urea 12.7
Glucose 16.5
PO_2 (air) 6.4 kPa
pH 7.29
Base excess -7.2.

A diagnosis of acute pancreatitis is made and this is predicted to be severe. The patient's age and past history increase the risks, so she is admitted to the HDU and a urinary catheter is inserted. Monitored oxygen therapy is commenced, an FiO_2 of 0.6 being required to keep the SaO_2 above 94%. The patient is fasted, and intravenous antibiotics are commenced.

Four hours later, the urine output tails off (<30 ml/h) despite a transient response to a further crystalloid fluid challenge. A central line is inserted and its position checked by CXR. Two more litres of crystalloid are needed over four hours to take the CVP to +7, at which level the urine output remains at 40 ml/h. The intravenous fluids are maintained at a rate of 4 l/24 h.

What would you do now?
An ultrasound scan shows gallstones in the gallbladder, mild dilation of the bile duct and a diffusely swollen pancreas. LFTs (serum bilirubin 35, alkaline phosphatase 230) suggest a degree of obstruction.

Urgent ERCP is arranged to exclude persisting biliary obstruction. The cholangiogram is normal.

The patient begins to improve, requiring less intravenous fluid to maintain urine output, and the FiO_2 is steadily reduced.

Learning points
- Often, the severity of an acute abdomen will become evident only over the hours following presentation – reassessment and changes to management will be needed.
- Patients with acute pancreatitis (and other conditions) sequester large volumes of tissue fluid around the inflamed pancreas during the hours after onset. Patients may continue to deteriorate rapidly into organ failure, but more of them respond to fluid, oxygen and other specific measures.
- A scoring system should be used for acute pancreatitis – patients predicted to have severe disease should be managed in the HDU according to established protocols.
- Any patient with an acute abdomen who needs high-flow oxygen or continuing fluid to maintain urine output is at high risk and needs a diagnosis, senior review, definitive treatment and a high level of care (HDU/ICU).

ASSESSING THE NEED FOR ICU/HDU ADMISSION

When you review a patient on the wards with an abdominal emergency or who has recently undergone major abdominal surgery, you need to be suspicious about the possibility of complications or the need to transfer the patient to a higher level of care. The onus is on you to be sure that the patient is progressing safely and satisfactorily, and in complex patients there may be many aspects to care across which they need to progress. Consequently, your assessment cannot be hurried, as it needs to be thorough and structured. The framework for assessment discussed in Chapter 2 will work for any patient. Table 9.1 shows some of the conditions about which you should be suspicious, and some further pointers are given below. If you are not sure whether the patient is stable, then they almost certainly are not and further assessment by senior surgical or ICU staff is needed. Call them but continue active assessment and management until they arrive.

Anticipate

Anticipate the need for ICU/HDU care from age, diagnosis, severity of the acute illness and presence of pre-existing diseases (see Table 9.2). It always pays to have considered this in advance and explored the availability of ICU/HDU support.

Table 9.2 *Anticipate the need for a higher level of care*

Age
Diagnosis
Comorbidity
Acute physiological status
Transfer to HDU/ICU prophylactically
Close monitoring to minimise delay in treating any
  complication

Deterioration

Deterioration in clinical signs should prompt immediate treatment and early intensive monitoring (see Table 9.3). Establish early and frequent monitoring of pulse, blood pressure, temperature and respiratory rate. Look carefully for trends of change, which may need early action. Urine output may need hourly monitoring with urinary catheterisation and CVP measurement to accurately manage fluid balance when appropriate. Patients who fail to progress also come into this category. This includes patients with apparently minor acute problems who do not respond rapidly to simple ward-type fluid resuscitation and also complex or elderly patients who fail to progress over a longer time course. Beware the surgical condition (*eg* anastomotic leakage) that presents initially as an ill-defined or medical diagnosis, otherwise the necessary surgical treatment may be delayed. Remember that even the best technical surgeons can have complications.

Table 9.3 *Detect and manage deterioration*

Resuscitate: ABCs
Transfer: safely and at appropriate stage (following discussion
  with the ICU and family)
Assess: patient, notes (especially op note/surgeon and
  comorbidity); consider other sources of information
Diagnose: clinically, investigate as needed, communicate with
  laboratory and radiology colleagues
Treat: is it surgical or medical? Consult and treat appropriately

Haematology

Beware the very low white cell count (neutropenia, $<2,000\times10^9/l$), which is a sign of profoundly impaired host response, and a raised count ($>20,000–25,000$), which is a sign of infarction. Beware anaemia, which may represent an undisclosed neoplasm or occult bleeding, sepsis or disseminated intravascular coagulation (DIC).

Biochemistry

Serum urea and creatinine values give a warning of dehydration or established renal failure. Blood gases may show the metabolic acidosis associated with tissue hypoperfusion and sepsis.

Blood cultures

Blood cultures are often negative in surgical infection and sepsis syndromes and may take 24–48 hours to give meaningful microbiological data. They may then give an idea of a source of sepsis, but they are of most value in guiding any adjustment of antibiotic therapy. This can be lifesaving; consequently, taking blood, urine and sputum cultures and culturing any pus or abdominal fluid are *mandatory* early steps.

Scoring system

The use of haematological, biochemical and clinical variables may be calculated into a scoring system such as APACHE II (used widely for all severely ill patients on ICU with a variety of disease processes), POSSUM (used for ward/HDU patients), or the Ranson or Imrie scores (used for acute pancreatitis). These offer comparative indices of disease severity but are of limited individual prognostic use. It may be appropriate to use them as one of several admission criteria to the HDU.

Imaging

Imaging with plain X-rays is rarely helpful, but early CT or ultrasound scanning may reveal a source of infection or sepsis and allow simultaneous active intervention, if a collection is seen, by percutaneous drainage. CT and particularly ultrasound can **miss** significant collections or pathologies, so although negative scans are a pointer they by no means exclude abdominal mischief. Positive scans should be acted upon. A Gastrografin enema or meal may help to define an anastomotic leak. Diagnostic peritoneal lavage or laparoscopy may be useful for an initial diagnosis of obscure acute abdomen in a sick patient (although impractical postoperatively), whereas a labelled leucocyte scan can be helpful in locating an obscure focus of infection when time is less pressing. Maintaining rapid progress towards a diagnosis and definitive treatment is essential in critically ill patients, and diagnostic laparotomy may be necessary (see below).

Case history 9.2

Six days after admission, you are called to review the patient with acute pancreatitis discussed in Case history 9.1. She had progressed well for 72 hours and had been discharged from the HDU to the general ward. Abnormal blood tests had started to return towards normal, but the patient had become reluctant to wear her oxygen mask continuously.

However, for the past three days, the patient had continued with low-grade abdominal pain and had not tolerated the restricted clear oral fluids that had been offered. The ward staff are now concerned that only 100 ml of urine has been produced in the last six hours. You reassess the patient and find her alert but in pain. She is tachypnoeic and dyspnoeic, has poor bibasal air entry and has basal dullness on percussion. Peripheral perfusion is poor, although blood pressure is normal. Heart rate is 98/min. JVP is not visible. The abdomen is distended and silent but only mildly tender deep in the epigastrium.

What would you do now?

What is your provisional diagnosis?

What tests (if any) would you request to establish the diagnosis?

You would administer high-flow oxygen and start a fluid challenge (10 ml/kg crystalloid). It is not clear whether the patient has deteriorated suddenly or whether the original process (pancreatitis) has continued unnoticed. Chart review shows that urea has fallen to 10.1 and white cell count (WCC) to 12.8 (last measured 36 hours ago), but neither have reached normal values. Intravenous fluids have continued through the CVP line at 3 l/24 h, although the CVP has not been measured since the patient

left the HDU. Since then, urine output has averaged only 800 ml/day. Taken with the pain and intolerance of oral fluids, it seems likely that the pancreatitis has continued at a more severe level than realised. Blood tests show the patient to be relatively hypoxic again and dehydrated, with a further increase in WCC:

    Haemoglobin 14.6
    WCC 18.9
    Amylase 72
    Sodium 131
    Potassium 3.9
    Urea 17.7
    Glucose 10.5
    PO_2 (FiO_2 0.6) 12.6 kPa
    pH 7.32
    Base excess − 2.3

The patient is clearly still unwell and is returned to the HDU. A CXR confirms bibasal collapse and shows small effusions, worse on the left, again typical of subphrenic pathology such as pancreatitis. The CVP is again measured and found to be low; fluids are adjusted accordingly.

This is one typical pattern for severe acute pancreatitis – to appear to improve only to relapse around the end of the first week. This is often related to pancreatic necrosis. You reassess two hours later: perfusion and urine output have improved following the fluid challenge and the patient is now well enough for definitive investigation by contrast-enhanced CT scan. This confirms necrosis involving 50% of the pancreas.

It is clear that the pancreatitis has some way to run. Nutritional support is needed and the options lie between nasojejunal feeding and parenteral nutrition. You elect to start total parenteral nutrition (TPN) through a dedicated arm of the CVP line and to introduce jejunal feeds slowly, as tolerated.

Learning points

- Severe pancreatitis often runs a protracted course – in this case, apparent improvement led to HDU discharge, but the medical follow-up on the ward was insufficient to detect a 'failure to progress' at the earliest stage. The same can occur with other abdominal conditions – structured reassessment and clinical suspicion are needed.
- Amylase remains acutely elevated for only 48 hours or so; after this, CRP provides a better index of the degree of persisting inflammation, although it is not specific to the pancreas.

- When a patient is unwell on the ward, they should be assessed and managed as intensively as if they presented through the emergency room.

SPECIFIC COMPLICATIONS IN SURGICAL CRITICAL CARE

Complications can occur after any operation, and the range is almost limitless. However, a few merit consideration here.

Anastomotic leakage

Anastomotic leakage is common (*eg* after 5–15% of colonic anastomoses). While signs may be obvious and typical, not infrequently they are **subtle** and **non-specific**. A high degree of suspicion, frequent reassessment and a low threshold for obtaining imaging studies are needed. Anastomotic leakage should be considered whenever there is unexplained postoperative deterioration. Certain patients are more at risk than others (see Table 9.4).

Table 9.4 *Risk factors for intestinal anastomotic leakage*

Anastomotic technique
  Tension, poor anatomical blood supply (particularly after anterior resection), unrecognised mesenteric vessel damage, poor suture technique (eversion or mismatch)
Local factors
  Obstruction, ischaemia or peritonitis
Systemic factors
  Shock (excessive bowel preparation or excessive blood loss), age, malnutrition, immunosuppression

The risk of leakage can be minimised by considering factors that influence anastomotic healing before, during and after surgery. Was perfusion during the operation compromised in any way? Was the patient shocked or dehydrated following bowel preparation (poor systemic perfusion is associated with poor visceral perfusion)? Were the vessels supplying the anastomosis inadequate (*eg* the blood supply to the splenic flexure is anatomically deficient)? Was there postoperative hypotension from any cause? When there are any risk factors, **anticipate** anastomotic leakage as a cause of poor recovery, a prolonged illness or signs of sepsis. Never let vanity delay having a second look at an anastomosis that might need exteriorisation or repair. In the critically

ill, when circumstances are otherwise unfavourable or when leakage has already occurred, it is safer to exteriorise suitable ends of small and large intestine than to attempt further anastomosis. There is also a place for ultrasound- or CT-guided percutaneous drainage for certain localised leaks and collections. If the patient's condition fails to improve, then reassessment with a view to further intervention is needed. Nutritional support is frequently needed.

Postoperative bleeding

Even in the presence of large drains, postoperative bleeding can be totally covert and there is always a considerable hidden proportion. Localised bleeding after surgery is usually technical in origin and often is surgically correctable by early intervention.

Primary haemorrhage occurs at operation. Certain sites are difficult to control – *eg* the pelvis and the injured liver – and may need packing. Packs need to be removed within 72 hours to prevent superadded infection and the risk of sepsis.

Reactive haemorrhage usually reveals itself in recovery (*eg* slipped ligature or aortic graft anastomotic leak) and needs early return to theatre for control. Patients who become overtly shocked almost always need surgery, as do patients who suffer a recurrence of lesser degrees of cardiovascular compromise, including fluid requirements that cannot be explained.

Secondary haemorrhage occurs seven to eight days postoperatively and is infection-related. This may be unheralded and unexpected, so control may be late and difficult to achieve. Proximal vascular control may be needed to stop the bleeding.

Patients with postoperative bleeding usually end up receiving a sizeable transfusion. This, together with the often-associated hypotension, coagulopathy and hypothermia, makes ICU admission advisable in many cases.

When more generalised signs (or sites) of bleeding occur, consider non-technical factors:

- anticoagulant therapy,
- recent large transfusion,
- sepsis and DIC, and
- unrecognised concomitant bleeding disorders, either congenital (*eg* Waldenström's macroglobulinaemia) or acquired (*eg* drugs).

In critically ill patients, coagulopathy is common and you may be asked to assess whether further surgery is needed. Correcting the coagulopathy is advisable before reoperating, but be careful about ascribing surgical bleeding to minor degrees of coagulopathy. Joint decision-making with the ICU staff helps. Coagulation ratios greater than 1.5 or so make surgery difficult.

Gastrointestinal stress ulceration (Curling and Cushing ulceration)

Nowadays, this is seen as a systemic disorder, being a reflection of systemic hypoperfusion. Ulceration and bleeding are increased in multiple organ dysfunction syndrome (MODS), and bleeding is more likely in the presence of a coagulopathy. For prophylaxis (*eg* in special risk cases such as burns, pancreatitis or uraemia) and treatment of established stress ulceration, cytoprotective agents such as sucralfate should be favoured. Histamine receptor or proton-pump antagonists increase gastric pH and favour bacterial colonisation. However, following oversewing of a perforated peptic ulcer (and in other patients with established peptic ulcer disease or therapy), proton-pump antagonists should still be used. There is usually a local policy to follow.

Venous thromboembolism

Pulmonary embolism (PE) remains a significant and all too frequent cause of death. DVT prophylaxis should not be forgotten in the critically ill, as their risk categorisation is high and thromboembolic deterrent (TED) stockings need to be supplemented with low-dose heparin and/or intermittent compression. Prophylactic measures should be routine in postoperative patients, and their use should be checked during the daily assessment.

In patients with a prior DVT/PE history, full anticoagulation should be considered but weighted carefully against other considerations. Similarly, patients with inherited thrombotic conditions (antithrombin III, factor V deficiency, protein C or S deficiency, etc) are not uncommon and will need careful management.

Clinical signs of DVT should be sought daily and followed up with duplex investigation in preference to diagnostic venography. Classic symptoms of PE occur in the minority of cases. Patients may simply have tachycardia and/or hypoxia; elderly patients may be confused or non-specifically unwell. In **unex-**

plained poor cardiopulmonary performance, exclude PE (which is commonly recognised for the first time at autopsy). In established repeated PE, a caval filter should be considered. Pulmonary angiograms or a spiral CT chest scan may be needed for the diagnosis of PE before thrombolysis or embolectomy in selected patients with cardiovascular compromise.

> **OPERATION NOTES**
>
> The findings at surgery and the procedure carried out are crucial in determining further management in all postoperative patients and all the more so in the sickest patients. The operation note communicates this information. Operation notes are often typed, but these take some time to reach the patient's notes, during which time adverse events may occur that need to be managed by staff not present at surgery. Essential findings, difficulties encountered, an outline of the procedure and clear postoperative instructions must be written out, particularly with regard to the management of drains, stomas and use of the gastrointestinal tract (see Fig. 9.1). Drawings of the arrangement of internal and external anatomy, drains and stomas are useful. This is particularly so when the patient is not being cared for on your usual surgical ward, eg on the ICU, and you may wish to supplement the note with an assessment of anticipated complications, particularly infective, or concerns about intestinal viability. It is the operating surgeon's responsibility to communicate clearly to their colleagues the need for any further planned intervention, eg removal of packs.

Necrotising fasciitis

Necrotising infection is life-threatening and must be recognised early. Immunocompromised patients who are diabetic, on steroids or having cancer therapy are particularly susceptible. Several eponyms (Meleney, Fournier) have been applied to rapid subdermal necrotising infection. These are caused by synergistic bacterial infection, in which several bacterial types create the conditions necessary for each other's growth. Gas may form in the tissues. Clostridial gas gangrene is less likely but is associated with severe systemic collapse; the degree of collapse can be very variable in other forms. Some patients exhibit relatively few clinical signs. Wide and courageous tissue excision to bleeding edges is needed, together with antibiotics and systemic support in order to save life or limb. All dead tissue must be excised if the process is to be controlled, and

LAPAROTOMY, SMALL BOWEL RESECTION, SPLENECTOMY
and HARTMANN'S PROCEDURE for ADVANCED
FAECAL PERITONITIS from DIVERTICULITIS.

MR LISTER

Perforated proximal sigmoid. Adherent small bowel
resected & anastomosed. Difficult to exteriorise colon
mobilised splenic flexure. Incidental splenectomy.
Full note dictated.

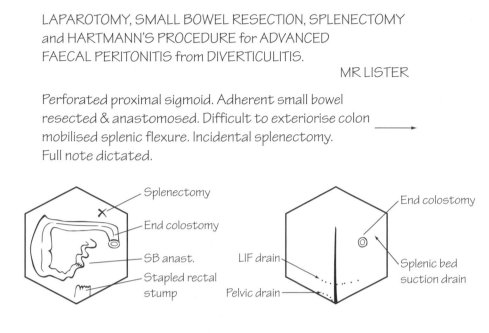

Postop:
- Nil by mouth & NG aspirates
- IVI to maintain urine output
- IV antibiotics (& ampicillin)
- Stoma care
- Drains – leave in place

- ICU support
- SC heparin
- TED stockings
- Pneumatic boots

Figure 9.1 *Operation note*

more than one operation is often needed. Skin grafts can be applied later.

Burst abdomen

Burst abdomen is largely a historical condition, since mass closure using non-absorbable (or delayed absorption) synthetic monofilament sutures is used nowadays. Usually, burst abdomen is heralded by the pink sign, a serosanguineous discharge eight to ten days after surgery (occasionally earlier). If there is prolapse of viscera, careful resuture or mesh insertion is needed. The immediate management is to keep the exposed viscera warm and moist with a sterile saline pack and to arrange for closure within three to four hours. There is usually little systemic upset immediately after the abdomen bursts, but the related overall mortality can be as high as 30%. In certain patients, a conservative management pol-

icy can be pursued when there is no skin rupture; an incisional hernia will result.

THE SURGEON IN THE ICU

The surgeon's involvement in hour-to-hour management in the ICU will vary between units, depending on the number and seniority of ICU staff. In any environment, the surgeon should remain completely informed about the patient's overall condition and vital organ function and should lead decisions about nutrition, drainage, use of the gut, and wound and stoma care. Although the ICU can be an unfamiliar environment, the surgeon must be responsible for the recognition and early treatment of persisting or secondary causes of acute abdomen. The surgeon has a vital role to play in the ICU as part of a multi-disciplinary team. Frequent review of surgical patients and prompt attendance when requested to assess other patients on the ICU is good surgical practice. Some surgical concepts and skills are outwith the many skills possessed by ICU staff and the surgeon should provide these and, in the longer term, any necessary educational input. Maintenance of a daily record of progress and management plans is as important in the ICU as in any other area of surgical practice.

Surgical input to ICU care on a twice-daily basis may help to recognise complications early, particularly those that require intervention. Persistent or worsening MODS requires a search for a source or factor (pus, leaked enteric content or dead tissue) to treat. In the face of sedation or paralysis, diagnosis is made more difficult and laparotomy should be considered. Atrial fibrillation may suggest embolic infarction in the gut or limb, but distinguishing between postoperative ileus and mechanical obstruction or infarction in such circumstances is particularly difficult.

Assessing the unstable patient on the ICU for abdominal pathology

Determining whether an unstable patient on the ICU has an abdominal process that requires intervention is a task that all doctors find difficult and one in which senior staff should play a major role. The same principles are used to assess complex patients on the HDU or on other wards; a patient with chronic renal failure with a possible acute surgical problem would be a typical example. As indicated above, this may be a **new complication** (eg acalculous cholecystitis in a patient with a head injury) or a **recurrent problem** (eg further sepsis in a patient with recent faecal peritonitis). Even in the latter case, there will usually be alternative sources of sepsis (chest, urine, lines, etc) that need quite different treatments with no less urgency. The stakes are high: missed significant abdominal sepsis in a patient with organ failure is almost always fatal. Likely problems can often be predicted from a knowledge of the patient's history.

Case history 9.3

Although the urine output of the patient encountered in Case histories 9.1 and 9.2 is maintained over the next 48 hours, saturations then fall steadily and the patient becomes increasingly tachypnoeic. An alert junior doctor makes contact with the ICU

for review before the patient tires and nears the point of respiratory arrest. An elective transfer to the ICU is arranged two hours later when a bed becomes available. However, following sedation, intubation and ventilation, urine output diminishes again and pulmonary artery catheterisation is necessary to guide inotrope therapy. You are asked to review the patient on the ICU and determine any need for surgical intervention.

Learning points

- Revise the indications for respiratory support and the relevant warning signs.
- Revise the manifestations of sepsis syndrome and its progression to organ failure.
- Any patient with abdominal pathology and organ dysfunction or failure needs urgent surgical review to establish a diagnosis and consider the need for intervention.

Patients with necrotising pancreatitis can deteriorate and develop organ failure for a number of reasons common to many critically ill patients, but the prime reason is because of infection of the necrotic pancreas. Patients with extensive necrosis, with unresponsive organ failure or who deteriorate are candidates for surgical necrosectomy, usually after guided fine-needle aspiration of the necrotic tissue to confirm the presence of infection.

You review the patient with your consultant, and a repeat CT with aspiration is arranged later the same day. CT shows that the necrosis has extended to involve 80% of the gland and microscopy shows bacteria in the aspirate. Once immediately stabilised, the patient is transferred to theatre for necrosectomy. The dead pancreatic tissue is removed and closed lesser sac lavage begun through four large drains. At the same time, a cholecystectomy, gastrostomy and feeding jejunostomy are carried out.

The first step is to make **your own full and thorough assessment** in the manner described earlier. After a preliminary discussion with ICU staff, you will need to review the charts, results and case notes (often sizeable) and examine the patient. Usual signs may be absent – sedation and paralysis will mask abdominal features – but other signs such as distension and the appearance of wounds, stomas and drain effluent may give clues. Frequently, the signs will be systemic, such as increased oxygen or ventilation requirements, increased inotrope requirements, onset of acute renal failure or thrombocytopenia. Almost any pattern of systemic deterioration can occur as a consequence of abdominal pathology. Although ICU care can often normalise the PaO_2 and blood pressure, it is the degree of ventilatory or inotropic support required to achieve these that varies and noting this is effectively your assessment of the ABCs in an ICU patient. Other usual pointers such as the white cell count may be less reliable, and often there will be confounding medical diseases or treatments (*eg* steroids). Previous radiology and operation notes are vital pointers, and sometimes it may be helpful to track down surgeons at other hospitals if the patient has been transferred to your hospital for ICU care.

DIFFICULTIES IN EVALUATING THE ABDOMEN IN ICU

Often, the signs are on the charts and not in the abdomen:

- Classic signs absent – look for worsening vital organ function:
    - ↑ O_2 required
    - ↑ inotrope needed
    - ↓ urine output.
- Clinical examination misleading.
- Mixture of medical diseases with new and old surgical problems.
- Investigation can be difficult to organise.
- Reoperation can be hazardous yet vital.

Often, the diagnostic question itself is simple and centres around the search for bleeding, perforation, dead bowel or sepsis, and the source of this. You will need to decide whether to rely on clinical judgement or whether radiological confirmation is needed. CT is usually the best means of imaging, but transferring ICU patients for CT is difficult and a rational analysis must be made of the risks and benefits of CT and the alternatives. Ultrasound is difficult and at times unreliable. Reoperative surgery carries higher risks and full exploration may be very difficult. CT can help localise areas of mischief, although it is by no means always accurate. If a sizeable abscess is seen on CT, you may decide that guided percutaneous drainage is appropriate; at times, this will be adequate. A failure to respond or incomplete drainage necessitates surgery.

Once you have evaluated the patient, you will need to discuss the case with your ICU colleagues again, as frequently alternative diagnoses are possible, each with differing treatment and risks. Line sepsis, urinary sepsis and pulmonary sepsis by bacteria or fungi should always be actively considered. Sometimes more than one cause may be contributing, and either over- or undertreatment can prove fatal. You may need to reassess key aspects together, but jointly you need to agree a cogent plan of investigation and action. The proposals can then be put to the relatives: the chances of death can be significant, and sometimes the relatives will feel that the patient has been through enough. As the investigations proceed, the patient's condition can be optimised for surgery; as with ward patients, the aim should be to operate in a timely manner on as well prepared a patient as possible. Often a balance is needed: it may not be possible to make the patient stable until the underlying cause is dealt with.

Case history 9.4

The patient seen in Case histories 9.1–9.3 stabilises on high-dose inotrope therapy, haemofiltration and pressure-controlled ventilation and then begins to improve very slowly. Jejunal feeding is tolerated. Closed lesser sac lavage continues.

Twelve days after the necrosectomy, the patient suddenly deteriorates again, becoming hypotensive and acidotic. Derived variables show the patient to be vasodilated. You are called to ICU to assess matters and confirm recent events. You find the patient's abdomen is cellulitic on the left side, and there is blood in one left-side drain and faeces in the other. The ICU nurse tells you that these drainages were clear yesterday. You discuss the position with the ICU team, who can find no other source of sepsis, the intravascular lines having been changed. You review the patient directly with your consultant and consider that a further CT will add nothing; it seems likely that the necrosis has progressed to involve the bowel, most usually the transverse colon. Together, your consultant and the ICU consultant explain to the family the balance between the difficulty and necessity of further intervention; the family accepts the advice that further surgery should be undertaken. At operation, further necrosis has spread down to involve the splenic flexure, which has perforated. The head of the pancreas and the adjacent colon remain spared. A transverse colectomy is carried out, together with a further necrosectomy, and the ends of the colon are exteriorised.

Despite further episodes of line sepsis, fungal superinfection and refractory diarrhoea requiring a return to TPN, the patient eventually recovers to leave the ICU for the HDU and then the ward. Six months later, you re-anastomose her colon.

Learning points

- Surgical complications occur on ICU and may need surgical management.
- Adequate treatment of the underlying cause of sepsis remains a vital principle.
- Signs of deterioration are different in the patient on the ICU, but the surgeon must be just as aware of them.
- Joint management offers the best chance of success.

A detailed account of the surgical techniques is beyond the scope of this book, but certain principles are shown in Table 9.5.

Table 9.5 *Principles of reoperative surgery for abdominal sepsis in the ICU patient*

Prepare the patient as well as is reasonably possible

Anticipate the difficulty of reoperative surgery – senior surgeon

Deal with the source of the problem definitively if at all possible

Exteriorise leaking bowel where possible

Remove dead tissue

Culture pus and drain sepsis

Consider gastrostomy or jejunostomy for ease of future management

When it has not been possible to excise all dead tissue or drain all sepsis, or where doubt exists about tissue (especially gut) viability, further surgery – a second look – may be employed at 24–72 hours to try to achieve these aims. The use of 'routine' repeat laparotomies is not of proven benefit and may cause harm. On occasion, it is not possible to close the abdominal wall without undue tension, and in such cases it may be necessary to leave the abdomen open with moist packing (known as a laparostomy) or with an inserted absorbable mesh to constrain the viscera. Any packing will need to be changed every 24 hours or so, and the surgeon should do this and re-lavage the abdomen on the ICU, if needed. If the underlying problem has been dealt with adequately, these open wounds heal remarkably quickly.

After emergency surgery (typically for aortic aneurysm, trauma or advanced peritonitis) or after the development of complications, the intra-abdominal pressure may rise due to visceral oedema. Once

the pressure is above 15 mmHg, progressive effects are seen on mesenteric, renal, pulmonary and ultimately cardiovascular function, a condition known as the abdominal compartment syndrome. Once at 25–30 mmHg, the patient will likely be anuric. If there is visceral compromise, then it may well be necessary to decompress the abdomen by leaving it open. The viscera are usually retained within a mesh or plastic bag that is sutured to the abdominal wound.

Abdominal-wall intestinal fistulae pose major challenges that may require HDU or ICU care for monitoring, fluid replacement and nutritional therapy, even in the absence of complicating infection or sepsis. There can be large losses of fluid and electrolytes with acid–base imbalance, particularly from high small bowel or duodenal fistulae, which need careful measurement with appropriate replacement and attention to nutritional support. The care of skin around fistulae is also skilled and requires the input of a stoma therapist. Dressings and bags can be tailored to protect the skin, and sump or other drains can assist collection of fistula fluid. The digestive action of certain fistulae (*eg* pancreatic) can add to infection and sepsis. When a patient develops a postoperative fistula, hasty reoperation can be harmful; it is often inappropriate to re-anastomose the bowel on account of sepsis and malnutrition. The Hope Hospital SNAP (sepsis, nutrition, anatomy, procedure) protocol can be used to good effect (see Table 9.6).

Table 9.6 *Approach to intestinal fistulae*

S	Sepsis	Drain adequately
		?CT-guided
		?surgery
		?defunction the bowel
N	Nutrition	Provide appropriately
		Often parenteral (see Chapter 12)
A	Anatomy	Define the site of the leak(s)
P	Procedure	Repair once the patient is well again, often after six months or so

The intact gut as a source of sepsis?

The importance of the intact gut as a source of sepsis in the ICU patient is debated. The gut is a rich potential source of bacteria and endotoxin, and the starved or hypoperfused gut may liberate factors into the circulation that might contribute to the organ dysfunction syndrome, especially following trauma.

After a few days of ventilation on the ICU, multiple trauma patients have a high risk of gut colonisation by bacteria, particularly aerobic Gram-negative bacilli. Without prophylaxis or active treatment, these bacteria contribute to a high mortality, mostly related to pneumonia, although urinary infections and soft-tissue infections are also common. The colonisation of the gastrointestinal tract is encouraged by intubation and by the use of histamine receptor antagonists or proton-pump antagonists. The raised gastric pH allows colonisation of the normally sterile upper gastrointestinal tract (which has been likened to an undrained abscess). Translocation of bacteria or other factors, macrophage stimulation, release of cytokines and promotion of ileus add to sepsis and intestinal failure, and hence add to difficulties with enteral nutrition.

Sucralfate is a gastric mucosal cytoprotective agent that keeps gastric pH low. Although reducing colonisation, it makes intestinal decompression difficult because it blocks the nasogastric tube. Problems with bacterial resistance may emerge. An attractive prophylactic measure is the early use of enteral feeding by fine-bore gastric or jejunostomy tubes. There appears to be no increased risk of anastomotic failure, and further advantage may be offered by the use of novel diets containing nucleic acids, polyunsaturated fatty acids and glutamine.

Stoma, drain and wound care on the ICU

STOMAS

Several stoma types may be needed on the ICU, and appropriate skill and teaching in management may fall to the surgeon who made them, together with a stoma care nurse.

Feeding gastrostomy or jejunostomy

A plan is needed for the start of stomal feeding and the amounts and types of nutrition in accordance with bowel function. Advice on when and how to remove the tubes may need to be passed on to ICU staff: 10 days is usually the minimum time allowed for a suitable seal to form before removal.

Faecal stomas

These may be temporary, loop or end-in type. Small bowel (ileostomy) effluent irritates the skin and usually a spout is made. A diverting loop ileostomy may cause difficulty in management (but is temporary). Large bowel effluent is more solid and is less irritant.

Two-piece stoma bag appliances minimise skin trauma in the early phase after surgery and maximise the chance of a skin seal being maintained. Once the skin is damaged, seek help from a skilled stoma therapist. Similar advice should be sought in caring for high-output fistulae, where expert techniques reap rewards. Patients who are conscious will also need psychological support once they realise they have a stoma. Nearby wounds need protection from faecal contamination in the early postoperative days.

DRAINS

Many drains are probably placed to ease the surgeon's mind after draining infection or to protect an anastomosis made in adverse circumstances. There is little evidence that they work efficiently beyond 24–48 hours. Drains may cause tissue reactions and persistent drainage. Whether closing dead space decreases the risk of complications or infection is open to doubt. Drains may be passive or may work by suction, and they may be open or have a closed (often with a one-way valve) collecting system. Most are of appreciable cost. Their indications may be debatable, but they are usually placed to 'protect' anastomoses (although they promote tissue collagenases) or to drain potential blood or other body fluid collections. They can be used for prolonged lavage, eg after laparotomy for pancreatitis, although their efficacy is debatable. The patency and function of suction drains can be improved and prolonged by using a sump drain (an inner tube under suction is protected from occlusion by a vented or irrigated outer tube). The surgeon will need to advise on volume of irrigation, etc. Underwater chest drainage is used specifically after chest trauma or surgery. It is appropriate for the operating surgeon to advise ICU staff on the management of drains, and how and when to remove them.

WOUNDS

In the UK, most wounds are closed primarily, even when they are contaminated. This is safe practice when the source of infection has been treated adequately and appropriate antibiotics have been given. In some circumstances, the skin of a laparotomy wound (eg after operation for faecal peritonitis), may be left open for delayed primary or secondary suture. The open skin wound is kept moist with saline or a very dilute aqueous antiseptic such as povidone–iodine or chlorhexidine, and when granulation tissue is established and clean (after four to five days) suture is followed by uncomplicated healing. This care of such wounds is the surgeon's responsibility. The same responsibility should not be overlooked on the ICU in deciding when sutures or clips should be removed. More complex wounds, such as those left after excision of necrotising infections or treatment of abdominal compartment syndrome, will require the surgeon to take a lead in the management and day-to-day debridement and irrigation.

SUMMARY

The abdominal viscera are a frequent source of sepsis and haemorrhage. Diagnosis may be difficult, particularly in the postoperative, sedated or paralysed patient, and there is no ideal radiological investigation to help manage all patients. Positive findings should be acted upon, and a high index of suspicion should be maintained in susceptible patients with negative clinical and radiological features. Diagnostic laparotomy may be needed occasionally. The aim is always to carry out necessary intervention **before** organ failure becomes established.

Communication, organisation and leadership in surgical critical care   **10**

Objectives

This chapter will help you to:

- Understand the importance of clear and effective communication in surgical critical care.
- Appreciate some of the barriers to communication and ways of overcoming these.
- Develop an increased awareness of the leadership role that the surgical registrar plays in the surgical team.
- Appreciate the value of personal and team organisation in facilitating leadership.
- Understand how people normally deal with adverse events and appreciate the frequency with which serious traumatic events can lead to stress reactions.
- Appreciate common psychological disorders in critical care and know when to refer to a psychiatrist.

Critical care involves many staff from a range of backgrounds who are called to work together – sometimes frequently, sometimes occasionally – under circumstances that are always pressurised and often stressful. For the critical care team to function at its best, and thereby stand any chance of delivering the best care consistently, there must be good communication and organisation. To achieve this, you need to understand some aspects of the ways in which people function under these circumstances, to learn to communicate better and to think about the ways in which you can contribute to the overall wellbeing of your team. Consider for a moment the range of communication skills, leadership skills and team skills that a successful surgical registrar may have to utilise during a busy weekend on call and you will quickly get an idea of the central role this topic plays in all of our practices (see Table 10.1). This chapter will deal with a few selected topics.

Table 10.1 *Communication skills and organisational issues typically used or encountered during a weekend on call*

Tasks/processes	Skills
Breaking bad news to patients or relatives*	Planning
Arranging investigations	Active listening
Ward rounds	Empathetic statements
Speaking to senior colleagues	Assertiveness
Speaking to junior colleagues	Avoiding aggressiveness
Speaking to multiprofessional team members	Use of silent pauses
Booking cases for operating theatre and ICU/HDU	Leadership
Coping with multiple jobs	Checking back
Dealing with emergencies	Summarising
Delegation and seeking help	Prioritising
Asking for help	

*This is a process rather than a single action/task

COMMUNICATION

> Communication matters – not just with the patient and relatives but also with colleagues.

It is important to be able to communicate effectively for many reasons:

- To elicit and to *provide information* quickly and accurately. Especially in the critical care setting, the quality and efficiency of this aspect of communication (data transmission) are important.

- To be able to *respond to emotional difficulties* in patients and relatives (empathy and emotional support). This may contribute to improved outcome and will improve satisfaction ratings and reduce complaints.
- To be aware of the possibility of *tension or distress building up* within the team and to know how to respond to this as your team will not work well when it carries this type of burden.

A comprehensive account of basic communication skills is outside the remit of this chapter, although certain relevant communication skills are discussed and practised on the CCrISP course. You should develop an awareness of basic communication skills, including the appropriate use of open, focused and closed questions, knowledge and avoidance of leading and multiple questions, and an understanding and use of empathetic statements (see Glossary at the end of this chapter).

What are the specific communication problems?

Surgical critical care frequently takes place in a setting in which background **obstacles** to communication are more likely. The patients are ill and frightened, and the staff are often over-busy but trying to perform to a high standard for clinical, ethical, moral and career reasons. At times of high emotion, there may be **impaired ability to concentrate** on the part of the patient, especially if there is pain, severe illness or complications of medication. Equally, operational **fatigue** on the part of staff is also important and may be hard to recognise. It is often easier for others to recognise the signs than the individual to identify these in themselves. Signs of operational fatigue include loss of clinical sharpness and a reduction in the quality of decision-making. This can cause particular problems at the top of hierarchical professions such as medicine. In addition, there may be irritability and anger, high tension, confusion (most obvious in organic brain syndromes, but may also occur in functional disorders), distress and tearfulness, and high expectations from patients and relatives and also from oneself and colleagues. Where the incident is a large-scale disaster, the scale of the event seems to amplify the impact. The media

may add to this effect, further stressing patients, families and staff.

Specific communication strategies

THE CRITICAL CARE SETTING

Communication strategies need to be **targeted** at the difficulties likely to be experienced. Critical care settings can be bewildering for patients and their relatives, often with a lot of strange high-technology equipment and sometimes with limited access to natural light. It is therefore especially important that **explanations** are provided at each stage. These can be simply to do with the role of a particular piece of equipment or an account of the next intervention. If it is an environment with limited natural light, this may increase disorientation, so readable clocks or other ways of helping to overcome this are important. Especially where there is a degree of organic confusion, aids to orientation can be important (*eg* photographs of loved ones). Easy-to-read name badges, primary nursing and other similar strategies can be helpful.

It may be necessary to repeat both questions and explanations at different times. Being prepared to go back over the history once the immediate crisis is over is good clinical practice and may turn up issues previously forgotten. Similarly, it is helpful to reduce fear by offering explanations more than once and using **check-backs** as a way of seeing how much the patient and relatives have really understood: often, it is hard to take it all in at first.

BREAKING BAD NEWS

The main communication issue is likely to be concerned with handling bad news. There is no perfect way to set out any communication process. What works well with some people in some situations can be a failure in others. However, some general principles are probably helpful.

The first principle is simply to *be prepared to talk* about bad news. The barriers to doing this may come from patients, or relatives if they are receiving the communication, or directly from ourselves. There are things that are hard for us to talk about, but in this setting it is important to be able to tackle some of these.

Attitudes have changed substantially in the last two decades, but the work of John Hinton in the

1970s with people who had terminal illnesses remains instructive. He found in an in-patient unit that, although staff believed that only a small minority of patients knew of their diagnosis and prognosis, a substantial majority had a very good understanding, *eg* through overhearing bedside conversations or through reading case files. The patients were able and willing to share this with Hinton in a way that they had not done with other staff. The most important point of this was that, when asked why they did not discuss their knowledge with staff, the patients often indicated that they did not want to cause the staff distress. In other words, patients chose silence partly to protect the staff working with them. From this, the concept arose of being prepared and able to give the patient *permission to talk* about bad news.

To be able to give permission effectively inevitably requires good listening skills. *Listening is an active process*, interspersed with signs of encouragement. We all do this differently, but through attitude, facial expression and verbal acknowledgements it involves showing interest and encouraging further disclosure.

The use of *empathetic statements* can be a straightforward way of identifying feelings and indicating support. These are statements in which the interviewer tries to identify a current feeling, such as sadness, anger or fear, and then ties it in to what has been happening: 'It sounds as if this news has made you feel more fearful than anything else.' This can allow the person to talk about their feelings, and it also gives the interviewer a chance to check whether what they perceive is correct. There are different ways of responding to sadness, anger and fear, for example. In contrast, sympathetic statements such as 'I know just how you feel' should be avoided since it is unlikely that you could feel the same and because they can lead to aggressive reactions in patients or relatives.

The most important aspects of helping people talk about their feelings are to allow time and space. The place should be quiet and (if talking to relatives or to mobile patients) private. The interviewer should give a sense of having time to talk. Often, it will not take much time (in general, more skilled communicators take less time than less skilled communicators), but it does require a little planning to ensure, for example, that discussions like this are not started a few seconds before a ward round or some other fixed event.

MEDICAL MISTAKES

Occasionally, people enter HDU care following a medical complication or even a medical error. This raises quite different communication issues. In addition to breaking bad news, there is the additional matter of handling feelings of guilt and fear of litigation. Again, it is not possible to make absolute statements, but in general, even in these situations, it is important to explain as fully as possible and, if an error has been made, to offer an apology. Not only is this in keeping with current thinking in the NHS but, since it is a sense of injustice that currently drives many into litigation, it is probably also a part of good risk management. It is important to be clear that one cannot apologise for the actions of others: you can state that you are sorry to hear of their concerns/worries and that they are entitled to a full reply to questions/complaints. It is dangerous to apologise for an event that occurs outwith the individual doctor's control (*ie* by another doctor or member of staff).

WORKING WITH COLLEAGUES

Staff relationships are of particular importance in critical care settings. Not only does the work involve vulnerable and dependent patients, but it also carries with it a lot of emotional issues to do with work with this group of people. It is easy for these pressures to translate into aggression and lack of respect. They may be made worse when interprofessional rivalries intervene or when people normally outside the unit are involved with particular patients.

Ideally, there needs to be some way for these issues to be dealt with on a team basis, such as identifying problem areas and finding supportive and effective ways of achieving change. Methods of achieving this cannot be prescribed but must vary with the precise situation. Deficient communication must be addressed in some manner, whether within or between professional groups and whether by individual or group meetings, formal or highly informal. These techniques often remain alien to the medical profession, but they can help greatly in the development of efficient and good-humoured units. Other ways open to individuals are to show respect in their own behaviour and to learn how to use assertive rather than either aggressive or passive ways of interacting (see Glossary at the end of this chapter). Sometimes, this is extremely difficult.

EVERYDAY COMMUNICATION IN SURGICAL CRITICAL CARE

Organisational skills

Surgical training covers basic knowledge, operative skills and, through courses such as the CCrISP course, guidance in practical management of acute conditions. Only infrequently do trainees receive advice or instruction about the organisation of their practice; regrettably, this is often discovered by each surgeon through a process that, to some degree, involves trial and error.

In any training programme, there is a point at which the surgical trainee begins to take increased responsibility for hour-to-hour management of unwell patients, to make critical decisions about the requirements for treatment of emergencies, and to carry out major and emergency operations as appropriate. This has been on promotion to the registrar grade in the UK; the name and stage at which this occurs will vary, but there is always a sizeable step up in the responsibility that the doctor carries. Of course, ultimate responsibility rests with the consultant in charge, but no surgeon can expect to carry out major procedures and not share in the responsibility for perioperative care.

Therefore, the specialist registrar will often be responsible for the daily business ward rounds, reporting as necessary to the consultant. It is unlikely that the consultant will make a formal ward round everyday, so it is essential that the registrar **actively** manages the patients, looks for and identifies problems, **makes decisions** about management and contacts the consultant if and when appropriate. Initially, registrars communicate very frequently with their seniors, but with training and experience the registrar's scope for safe practice can and should expand.

For critical care to be delivered successfully in the context of a busy surgical practice, many things need to happen during the course of the day – different facets of care, investigations, decisions, investigations and operations. These do not happen automatically. As a registrar, you have to learn to conduct this orchestra of activity, which is not always an easy task. To achieve success, you will need to organise yourself (and sometimes others), exercise a degree of leadership, communicate effectively and become able to make decisions.

To make decisions, you need information, and you get this from communication. As you train, you need to become aware of what information you do need and what information is largely superfluous to any critical decision. There is a balance to be struck between hasty and unfounded decision-making and unnecessary delay waiting for tests that will add little or nothing. Getting information takes you or others time, and you need to delegate and organise appropriately. To be efficient, you need to timetable your business ward rounds such that key information is most likely to be readily available from nurses and house staff. You need to be prepared to circumvent blocks to your patients' progress. It may prove difficult to get old notes, get a certain test or opinion, or administer a certain drug. At times, you will need to be quite assertive on your patients' behalf to get what they need, but you need to learn when to be assertive and when the thing you cannot get will not really make any difference to care.

> Organise to make communication easy and rapid.

To get the best out of a team, leadership is required. This requires a range of skills, including ability, knowledge, personality, decision-making, appropriate humour, humility, acceptance of others' views and firmness. All must be deployed at the right time, and few if any of us possess all or even a majority of these attributes. You will need to work hard, praise and support your colleagues, admit when you are wrong or don't know, and get timely help. Dealing with seniors is a whole skill in itself. Few consultants will not wish to be informed promptly about unwell patients, but all will expect you to have assessed the patient, begun immediate treatment and arrived at some decisions, including a provisional plan of action. The exception to this is the patient who clearly needs an immediate operation beyond your ability – *eg* a collapsed patient with penetrating trauma – in which case, the consultant will want a brief, clear message and will probably give you a brief, clear reply.

Clinically, you will need to lead by example: if you are not thorough, why will anyone else be? Reassessing patients is probably the single most neglected skill – clinical patterns will emerge and diagnoses become obvious. Utilise the support services available – good and experienced nurses have an enormous amount of help they can give you, particularly about how unwell a patient is.

Managing emergencies and deciding on the need for urgent surgery is difficult. Patients need a diagnosis, and unstable patients need a **diagnosis and treatment** urgently. Regrettably, patients do not improve magically between 2am and the 8am ward round: the emergency patient who fails to respond to simple resuscitation in the middle of the night needs a plan of action-making then. This may involve conservative or operative treatment, but lack of knowledge or an inability to conduct a particular operation is **never** an adequate reason for delay. Decision-making is active, not passive.

Continuity of care is essential for patients' wellbeing in critical illness. Junior doctors' hours have changed, but the need has not: the onus is now on the 'owning' team to pass on problems to the duty team, but also on the duty team to look for problems among the patients of all the surgical teams and to deal with them promptly.

Becoming a registrar is a stressful but enormously rewarding time. You will very quickly develop new operative and patient management skills and begin to feel that you really are a surgeon. Organise yourself and your practice, and communicate and listen effectively to make the learning process less stressful for all.

COPING WITH ADVERSE EVENTS

Emotionally charged events are common in everyday life and particularly so in the critical care setting. This holds true for relatives and staff, as well as for patients. Coming to terms with these everyday events is a largely automatic process. In simple terms, it seems to include having an awareness of the emotional reaction and somehow returning towards a normal balance. Traumatic stressors are events that act upon people to produce intense pressure or tension; they are associated with the negative emotions of fear and sadness. In normal circumstances, these emotional reactions decline gradually, and each subsequent recall of these feelings is rather less intense until eventually, as a new equilibrium is reached, the emotional reaction fades completely as the individual adapts.

Faced with events that are perceived to be especially traumatic, this adaptive mechanism may be overwhelmed. The initial emotional reaction may be so intense that the only viable reaction is to attempt to prevent or avoid (blot out) these painful feelings.

This may be achieved by avoiding places or objects that remind the person about the trauma, or through suppression of emotions in general – 'emotional numbing'.

These defensive reactions will rarely be completely successful, and the individual is left with painful intrusive recollections that alternate with defensive avoidance. This cyclical reaction of intrusion and avoidance is the central element of post-traumatic stress disorder (PTSD). It is possible that as the emotions are suppressed, because they are too extreme, they are not held in awareness and do not decline. The condition becomes chronic and may be frankly disabling. Stress disorders are not rare: some symptoms of PTSD are seen in the majority of patients who are involved in significant accidents, and features occur in relatives of the victims and also in staff. Typically, patients may report recurrent and intrusive distressing recollections of the event, including flashback episodes. These can be precipitated by cues that symbolise or resemble an aspect of the traumatic event (*eg* hearing a car's brakes on TV or even driving past the hospital). The victim is likely to avoid thoughts or cues that activate memories of the event and may become withdrawn or detached or appear depressed.

Critical events are a significant cause of occupational stress for staff groups (including doctors) in this environment, and this is important to recognise not only for personal and team wellbeing but also because operational fatigue and impaired performance may result. **Awareness** of stress reactions is the first step, and the provision of appropriate support of colleagues and patients, largely through opportunities for discussion, will represent a significant advance in many settings. The initial aim is to provide a means for people to talk about a critical event, learning about some of the ways that people may respond and (usually) achieving an understanding that their own behaviour is within a normal range.

COMMON PSYCHOLOGICAL DISORDERS IN SURGICAL CRITICAL CARE

So far, the emphasis has been on specific reactions to adversity, but of course a wide range of problems may occur. Traumatic life events may trigger feelings of depression, anxiety or even relapse of certain psychoses. Thus, the assessment needs to cover the full range of psychological difficulties. In this section, brief reference will be made to four of these.

Anxiety

Mild feelings of fear, apprehension, sadness and emotional turmoil are very common in anyone admitted to hospital with a serious condition. In general, the **approach taken by the clinical team** can often determine the amount of distress experienced. A team that works together well, communicates well with patients and offers appropriate emotional support will stand to reduce these difficulties. Of course, the opposite is also true.

Assessment is likely to centre on asking appropriate questions about current feelings and enquiring into any associated autonomic symptoms of anxiety (*eg* tachycardia) that may mislead in the assessment of physical health. Sometimes, visible overbreathing (excessive, often irregular breathing) may be a clue to the presence of the chronic hyperventilation syndrome. This can present with a multitude of physical symptoms and is often associated with anxiety or depression.

Major depression

Depression is a common, often unrecognised condition. It spans a wide range of severities and patterns of reaction. The core feature is a depressed mood, in which there is loss of pleasure and enjoyment, reduced interest, hopelessness and helplessness, and pessimism for the future. In addition, there are often biological features, such as loss of weight, impaired sleep with early morning wakening, and a diurnal variation of mood, being worst in the early morning. Finally, there may be evidence of a frank psychosis, with mood-congruent delusions and hallucinations. These may include delusions of worthlessness or guilt, delusions of cancer, delusions of persecution (felt to be deserved) and accusatory auditory hallucinations. All these are in keeping with the primary disturbance of mood.

As a routine in the assessment of psychiatric disturbance, there should be an investigation of **suicidal thinking**. One of the ways of asking about this is to combine a permissions statement with questions. For example, 'If someone has talked about feeling very unhappy, they sometimes cannot see much point in life.' Then continue with something like 'I wonder if you have ever felt that it would be better just to go to sleep and never wake up?' This can be followed by further questions about any suicidal thoughts, any suicidal plans (going into detail if needed) and any suicidal behaviour. In this way, the whole subject can be covered easily without causing excessive concern. There is no excuse for failing to ask about suicidal thinking in the presence of significant psychiatric disturbance.

Alcohol dependence

This is included as a reminder that alcohol problems are common (in general, about one in five people in hospital have significant alcohol-related problems) and can cause complications in the critical care setting. The characteristic problem arises from withdrawal symptoms, which follow hospitalisation and enforced abstinence. These can include typical tremor, nausea and mood disturbances, but may extend to delirium tremens and even convulsions.

Acute organic reactions

Variously styled as confusional states, toxic confusional states, deliriums, etc, these are short-lived organic disturbances characterised by confusion, clouding of consciousness (sometimes quiet subtle), disorientation and often marked fearfulness. There may be delusions, often persecutory. Common causes include alcohol withdrawal and prescribed medication (*eg* analgesia), but they may also occur in the context of a wide range of medical conditions. Following assessment and correction of the ABCDs of the initial assessment, further evaluation is centred on the cognitive state – ability to attend and retrieve, awareness of environment, etc – and on the possible causes that also require full assessment. This is an organic disorder in the psychiatric classification because it is always secondary to some physical dysfunction. It is likely to be made worse by a disorienting environment and by a failure to offer frequent and repeated explanations.

When to refer to a psychiatrist?

To some degree, this depends on the capacity and engagement of the local psychiatric service. However, there are clear indicators for referral, which are important to outline. First, there is the situation where the diagnosis is uncertain and especially where there may be a psychiatric component. Somatisation disorder and Munchausen's syndrome are extreme examples, but there are often complex interactions between physical and psychological processes that may require assessment. It is important in these situations to make positive psychiatric assessments rather than assumptions based on the absence of signs of physical disorder.

There are situations in which either the **severity** of the psychiatric condition or the level of **danger** associated with the condition make referral both appropriate and often urgent. This might be the case following, for example, deliberate self-harm or the development of persecutory beliefs in an acute organic reaction leading to thoughts of murder.

One situation in which referral is often considered is in relation to consent. Psychiatrists have special knowledge of the legislation concerning consent to treatment for psychiatric illness. The relevant legislation has much less to say about consent to treatment for physical illness, and common law principles usually apply. None the less, as long as a referral is not made with overoptimistic expectations, it may still be useful to discuss difficult cases where consent is withheld as this is an issue that is more common in psychiatric practice.

CONCLUSIONS

This chapter cannot provide a comprehensive account of the field but perhaps it will help to highlight those areas where further learning is required. Communication skills are especially important as they help to make practice more **effective** and more efficient. More can be achieved in less time. It is important to look at patients, relatives and staff groups and understand the ways in which we cope with the everyday workload and adversity and how these mechanisms can be overwhelmed at times of crisis.

GLOSSARY

Most clinicians could improve their communication skills, and surgeons are certainly no exception. The two parts of this glossary outline some principles about which you may wish to read further.

Basic communication skills

In this section, some of the terminology is explained. It is useful in data-gathering to use an appropriate range of open, focused and closed questions. In taking a history, the open question 'Is there anything else?' is useful as a final question.

Open questions can take a wide range of responses, *eg* 'What is the main problem?'

Focused questions can take a limited range of responses, *eg* 'Which is the worst pain today?'

Closed questions must be answered 'yes' or 'no', *eg* 'Is the pain in the knee the worst pain that you have had?'

Some questions are likely to produce misleading answers. A leading question expects a particular response, and this may be given even if it is wrong. Multiple questions are common in checklist approaches to the history, but the answer given may relate only to the final item in the list; again, this is misleading.

A *leading question* expects a particular answer, *eg* 'The pain is worst at night, isn't it?'

Multiple questions include a list, *eg* 'Do you have problems with chest pain, shortness of breath or ankle swelling?' This might attract the answer 'No', which to the patient might be 'no' only to ankle swelling but to the doctor might be 'no' to the three items together.

There is a skill to *checking back* – being prepared to check that you have the right understanding – or using a *summary* of the main features as a way of confirming the history with your patient.

There is also a skill to *sharing a problem*. If you do not know how to handle something in an interview, sometimes the best thing is to own up, *eg* 'I have a feeling that you are upset but I am not sure what has caused it. Is it OK to ask you about it?' or 'My problem is that I have only five minutes before I have to go to theatre. I really need to ask you about something. Is that alright?'

Finally, perhaps the most useful of the active steps in understanding emotional reactions is the *empathic comment*. This is a statement identifying an emotional reaction, *eg* 'That must have made you feel very frightened.'

In making this statement, a lot of care must be exercised to listen to what is being said and not simply to assume that everyone will experience fear, anger, sadness, *etc*, in specific situations. It is useful as a way of checking back on emotions; more importantly, it communicates that you can appreciate at least some of what your patient is feeling. This can be a very powerful intervention and should be a skill available to all doctors.

Assertiveness, passivity and aggression

In being assertive, communication allows each person to express their honest opinions without needlessly hurting the other person.

In being passive, honest opinions are suppressed.

Aggression involves the use of excessive force or power causing needless suffering. This can be active aggression (*eg* violent, insulting speech) or passive aggression (*eg* emotional manipulation).

Assertiveness is therefore usually the preferred option. In general, assertive statements contain the pronoun 'I', whereas aggressive statements more often include the pronoun 'you', *eg* 'I feel that the patient would be better helped by this approach' versus 'You are incompetent and have got this all wrong'.

The specific skills cannot be summarised in a short glossary but are included in most books on communication.

Objectives

This chapter will help you to:

- Be aware of the frequency, causes and importance of inadequate nutrition among critically ill surgical patients.
- Understand the metabolic responses to starvation, injury and sepsis and the implications of these responses for the provision of nutritional support.
- Know how to assess nutritional status and devise

regimens for nutritional support comprising macronutrients, trace elements, vitamins and minerals.
- Be able to assess the most appropriate route for the administration of nutritional support.
- Be able to recognise and manage the complications associated with nutritional intervention.

BACKGROUND

Malnutrition is a **common** finding in surgical patients. As many as 50% of patients on general surgical wards are reported to exhibit signs of protein–energy malnutrition (PEM), and its relevance to outcome has been well established. More than 60 years ago, loss of more than 20% of preoperative weight was shown to increase the mortality associated with gastrectomy for benign disease 10-fold. Similar figures have been produced for morbidity and mortality in patients undergoing surgery for a wide variety of malignant and benign conditions. Although in many cases these effects may be due to the nature of the disease process itself rather than malnutrition, it is important to ensure that, wherever possible, inadequate nutritional intake does not add to the likelihood of a poor outcome in critically ill and postoperative patients.

In many critically ill patients (notably those with the systemic inflammatory response syndrome (SIRS) and sepsis), the underlying problem relates to **impaired utilisation** of fuel substrates, rather than deficiency, and no amount of externally added nutrients will reverse the process that is consuming the body's reserves. Efforts must be directed therefore to the **underlying cause** (eg seeking and

draining infection or removing dead tissue). Even in patients with simple starvation, nutritional support needs to be given for a minimum of two weeks preoperatively before any significant benefit can be anticipated. While the morbidity associated with starvation should not be added to a patient who is already sick, it is important to be guarded in our expectations of the benefits of nutritional therapy. Nutritional support should be considered for **every** surgical patient unable to resume adequate dietary intake for more than three or four days and in every critically ill patient, although its benefit may not be realised until the underlying disease process abates.

Although naso-enteric feeding has been practised since 1598 and feeding jejunostomy was described over 100 years ago, the most significant advances in the nutritional management of surgical patients occurred in the 1930s and 1940s, at a time when the metabolic response to starvation, injury and sepsis was starting to be understood. These advances were associated with development of the technology for the delivery of parenteral nutrition, an appreciation of the requirements for glucose, lipid and amino acids in nutrient mixtures, and later recognition of the importance of trace elements, vitamins and minerals.

The importance of nutritional support in surgical patients is now recognised widely, but the financial cost is potentially enormous: recent estimates for parenteral nutritional support reached almost $3200/patient in the USA. The costs were found to be highest in patients felt least likely to benefit. Cost-effective delivery of nutritional support requires an understanding of the associated indications, techniques and complications, while an appreciation of nutritional requirements of the critically ill patient requires an understanding of the metabolic environment in which nutritional support is to occur.

METABOLIC RESPONSES TO STARVATION, INJURY AND SEPSIS

Occasionally, surgical malnutrition is simply starvation due to fasting (whether necessary or otherwise), but surgery and sepsis cause a **systemic metabolic response** that contributes very significantly to the clinical picture and to nutritional management.

Feeding and fasting

In health, feeding replenishes fuel stores and the oxidative metabolism of fuel generates energy for metabolic processes. The normal daily resting energy expenditure of a 70-kg man is approximately **1,800 kcal**. The brain uses carbohydrate as its sole fuel in the fed state and requires approximately 100 g of glucose each day. Any glucose not consumed by the brain is used to restore liver carbohydrate stores (glycogenesis) and the rest is converted to fat (lipogenesis).

Amino acids are used to replenish those lost in the normal daily turnover of protein (including skeletal and cardiac muscle, liver and intestinal structural proteins, and liver export proteins such as albumin), while the rest are metabolised in the liver, which converts the carbohydrate component into fuel (gluconeogenesis) and the nitrogenous component to urea for excretion.

Lipid is stored primarily as triglyceride within adipose tissue. Lipid cannot be converted directly into either amino acids or glucose.

The hormonal environment associated with recent feeding (high insulin levels and low glucagon levels) allows the storage of nutrient described above.

After a short (12-hour) fast, all the food ingested during the previous meal is likely to have been used. Plasma insulin levels are low and plasma glucagon levels are rising. The major source of glucose for the brain is now from the glycogen stored in the liver (of which there is approximately 200 g). This breakdown of muscle glycogen to provide glucose (glycogenolysis) is also facilitated by these hormonal changes. Skeletal muscle contains a much greater amount of glycogen (500 g), but this glycogen cannot contribute directly to the provision of glucose for other tissues. Instead, glucose is converted to lactate within muscle, and the lactate is exported to the liver for conversion to glucose (Cori cycle). Glucose is also converted to lactate within haematopoietic tissues.

Muscle tissue derives approximately one-third of its energy from the oxidation of glucose and the rest from the oxidation of fatty acids derived from the breakdown of fat in adipose tissue (lipolysis). Muscle protein breakdown begins to contribute amino acids (alanine and glutamine) for the formation of glucose in the liver and, to a lesser extent, the kidney.

After about 48 hours of starvation, approximately 75 g of muscle protein is being broken down each day. This provides precursors for hepatic gluconeogenesis. Glycerol and triglycerides from the fat depots are being used to make up the shortfall in energy requirements, and fatty acids provide the main metabolic fuel for many tissues.

With more prolonged fasting, a series of metabolic adjustments develop in order to preserve body protein (see Table 11.1). The most important adaptation (and one that is conspicuous by its absence in critical illness) concerns the gradual increase in the capacity of the liver to produce acetoacetate and beta-hydroxybutyrate (ketone bodies) from fatty acids. The brain adapts to use these, thereby reducing the need for muscle breakdown by up to 55 g/day. This adaptive ketogenesis preserves vital muscle and visceral protein and persists as long as ketone body production persists, fuelled by the availability of fat stores. While absolute rates of protein breakdown decrease (in contrast to critical illness), the reduced anabolism that results from the lack of substrate leads to a net catabolism. These metabolic adjustments are associated with low levels of insulin and high plasma glucagon concentrations. A gradual decline in the conversion of inactive thyroxine (T_4) to active tri-iodothyronine (T_3) results in a fall in energy requirements to approximately 1,500 kcal/day.

Table 11.1 *Metabolic responses to fasting*

Insulin levels fall
Glucagon levels rise
Hepatic glycogenolysis
Muscle and visceral protein catabolism
Hepatic gluconeogenesis
Lipolysis
Ketogenesis, sparing 55 g/day of muscle protein
Fall in metabolic rate (typically to 1,500 kcal/day)

Metabolic responses to injury (including surgery)

After injury, whether accidental or surgical, there is a modified metabolic and clinical response (see Table 11.2). Many of the metabolic responses to injury can be understood on the basis of the associated hormonal alterations. Release of noradrenaline, adrenaline, glucagon, growth hormone and cortisol (the so-called 'counter-regulatory hormones') occurs. Initially, plasma insulin levels fall, but later they may rise to levels in excess of those normally encountered for a given glucose concentration. The normal anabolic effects of insulin are impaired (**insulin resistance**). In addition, there is a relative increase in glucagon concentration. The hormone response increases with the severity of trauma, its effect being to **increase the availability of fuel** for metabolic processes.

Table 11.2 *Metabolic responses to injury*

Modest rise in metabolic rate and therefore energy expenditure (typically 2,000 kcal/day)
'Counter-regulatory' hormone response: adrenaline, noradrenaline, cortisol, glucagon and growth hormone
Resistance of tissues to effects of insulin
Glucose intolerance
Preferential use of lipid as energy source
Exaggerated gluconeogenesis and breakdown of muscle protein, despite feeding
Loss of adaptive ketogenesis

There is a modest increase in the metabolic rate to approximately 2,000 kcal/day. Muscle protein breakdown increases, and glycogenolysis and gluconeogenesis result in an increased availability of glucose, but **lipid** appears to be the major fuel used for energy production after injury. The extra glucose produced is instead used primarily by the brain, white blood cells and the healing wound. There is continued release of amino acids from muscle to provide gluconeogenic precursors (particularly alanine). Glutamine is also released from skeletal muscle and under conditions of stress appears to be essential for the normal functioning of cells in the small intestine and immune system. Alanine and glutamine are formed within skeletal muscle from the metabolism of a special group of essential amino acids called branched-chain amino acids (BCAAs leucine, isoleucine, valine), which can be taken up by muscle cells. The adaptive ketogenic, protein-sparing response described above does not occur as long as there is insulin resistance.

As the stress response wanes and insulin resistance abates, the patient becomes capable of making up the lost reserves of protein and energy (*ie* anabolism supervenes). This usually coincides with the resumption of eating and of increasing mobility (muscular exercise), both of which are required to restore muscle mass.

Metabolic responses to sepsis and the systemic inflammatory response syndrome

The changes in metabolism that develop with the onset of sepsis/SIRS are complex and represent an exaggeration of those described after injury (see Table 11.3). The key changes are a markedly increased metabolic rate (**hypermetabolism**) and rate of **protein breakdown**. There may be marked glucose intolerance, with the development of a 'diabetes-like' state. Despite this hyperglycaemia, glucose utilisation and storage are impaired and the septic patient has a greater reliance upon fat as a metabolic fuel for energy production. There is frequently marked fluid retention and up to 20 l of water may be retained within the tissues of the critically ill patient because of significant increases in microvascular permeability, compared with 1–2 l seen after major surgery. The rate of protein breakdown may reach 250 g/day; muscle and visceral protein is thus consumed for the generation of glucose, despite the frequently elevated plasma glucose concentration. Although some of this exaggerated muscle protein breakdown might be due to the hormonal environment, the release of cytokines such as interleukin-1, interleukin-6 and tumour necrosis factor (TNF) may also play a part.

Table 11.3 *Metabolic responses to sepsis/SIRS*

More marked increase in metabolic rate and therefore energy expenditure (2,200–2,500 kcal/day)

Exaggerated gluconeogenesis, protein catabolism and muscle wasting

Marked fluid retention

Insulin resistance is common and may be severe

NUTRITIONAL ASSESSMENT

PEM often goes unrecognised in surgical patients, despite its frequency and its adverse prognostic implications. An assessment of the patient's nutritional status should form part of the physical examination. Gross degrees of malnutrition manifest as obvious wasting are recognised easily, but more subtle degrees of deficit may not be, particularly in the obese patient. Studies utilising accurate methods of assessing body composition (such as in vivo neutron activation analysis, IVNAA) have shown how common depletion of protein is; they have also shown that many of the traditional methods of assessment are highly unreliable. If any commonly available objective measure of nutritional status is to be used, then body weight is probably still the most useful. Weight (in kilograms) should be standardized to the square of the height (in m²) to allow for calculation of the body mass index (BMI). A history of recent weight loss is also of particular importance. A BMI of less than 18.5 and/or unexplained recent (within the last six months) loss of more than 10% of body weight usually indicates a patient at high risk of undernutrition.

Anthropometric measurements (*eg* measures of skinfold thickness and mid-arm circumference) to allow estimation of muscle mass (protein reserves) and fat mass (energy reserves) may be of value in population studies, in healthy individuals and in patients with simple malnutrition, but measurements using these techniques are unlikely to be accurate in individual patients, particularly if they are critically ill. Functional tests, including handgrip and respiratory muscle strength, are predictive of the loss of muscle mass but have limited clinical applicability.

Formulas to assess energy requirements such as the Harris–Benedict equation rely on poorly substantiated 'correction factors' for various clinical conditions such as sepsis or burns and tend to overestimate energy expenditure. The most accurate way (albeit still with substantial variability) to assess energy expenditure in the clinical setting is by indirect calorimetry, using a bedside 'metabolic cart'. This technique, which involves measurement of oxygen consumption and CO_2 production requires expensive equipment and is generally beyond routine clinical use.

Laboratory tests that are claimed to reflect malnutrition range from the simple, such as albumin, prealbumin and total lymphocyte count, to the complex, including assessment of cell-mediated immunity and lymphocyte responses to mitogens. These investigations, however, principally measure how 'sick' the patient is and are surrogate measures of the severity of the process that has led to malnutrition rather than measures of inadequate nutritional intake per se. For example, in simple starvation, serum albumin concentrations remain unaltered for nearly six weeks and begin to fall just before death. In contrast, in sepsis, the serum albumin concentration commonly falls to below 20 g/l within a couple of days or even hours, principally due to redistribution into the interstitial space.

Laboratory investigations to look for the presence of associated trace element, vitamin and electrolyte deficiencies, however, may be of value. Measurement of standard electrolytes along with magnesium, calcium and phosphate will enable demonstration of major electrolyte abnormalities. Interpretation of sodium and potassium balance may be exceptionally difficult in critically ill patients, especially in the presence of large gastrointestinal losses (*eg* in association with an intestinal fistula or a proximal stoma). Under these circumstances, estimation of 24-hour urinary electrolyte output may be of value. Estimation of urinary nitrogen output is rarely of clinical value. Other laboratory investigations for detection of specific deficiencies, where the clinical history suggests prolonged inadequate intake, include prothrombin time/international normalised ratio (INR) (indicating vitamin K status, assuming normal liver function), red cell indices (vitamin B_{12}, folate). Low serum zinc concentrations may be indicative of deficiency, but because zinc is transported bound to albumin, levels tend to fall with hypoalbuminaemia.

While an assessment of the degree of metabolic stress to which the patient is being subjected can be made, the most important step in nutritional assessment is to **consider the need** for nutritional support in every patient based upon underlying diagnosis, recent events and the likely time to restoration of adequate nutritional intake. Adequate nutritional intake does **not** occur automatically when the patient is first allowed to commence oral fluids.

PROVISION OF REQUIREMENTS

The need for water, electrolytes and nutrients in healthy subjects has been well defined, but the effects of differing disease processes upon these requirements are, in many cases, unclear. Estimation of an individual's requirements for nutrients, fluid and electrolytes should take place at the same time as other aspects of drug therapy are reviewed.

In the case of fluid and electrolytes, daily estimation of requirements should be performed. In patients with a high-output stoma or fistula, twice-daily estimation of requirements together with assessment of balance are needed.

Nutrient requirements are liable to much slower changes and twice-weekly assessment is generally sufficient. Review of whether nutrient requirements are being met is conducted at the time of nutritional assessment (see above).

Water and electrolytes

Water requirements in the critically ill patient are subject to much wider variations than in healthy subjects. In the latter case, 2–2.5 l of water each day will usually meet basal requirements. In critically ill patients, major **gastrointestinal** losses of water and electrolytes and **insensible** losses of water associated with evaporation from open wounds and the respiratory tract may add significantly to requirements. **Sequestration** of water (up to 20 l) within tissues as a result of increased capillary permeability and hypoalbuminaemia, together with impaired renal homeostatic function, may complicate the assessment of water requirements. Starting points are as follows:

- *Children:*
  - 100 ml/kg/day for first 10 kg body weight
  - 50 ml/kg/day for next 10 kg body weight
  - 25 ml/kg/day for each subsequent 1 kg body weight
- *Adults:* 30 ml/kg/day

Requirements of electrolytes vary greatly according to the clinical state of the patient. In health, the 70-kg adult requires approximately 100 mmol of sodium and 60 mmol of potassium each day. Provision of these amounts will maintain electrolyte balance in patients unable to take oral fluid and without pathological losses. Critically ill patients frequently have electrolyte requirements in excess of those seen in health.

Patients with gastrointestinal fluid losses in excess of 1 l will generally require intravenous fluid therapy, and these losses should be replaced by amending the electrolyte content of the feeding regimen appropriately. A useful simple rule is to replace gastrointestinal losses millilitre for millilitre as Ringer's lactate.

Potassium deficiency may be profound despite apparently normal serum potassium concentration, since the vast bulk of exchangeable potassium (3,500 mmol) in the body is intracellular and only about 70 mmol is in extracellular fluid. Replacement of potassium may lead to temporary restoration of serum potassium, which then repeatedly declines as equilibration occurs. Other factors that influence electrochemical balance across membranes (*eg* acidosis) may alter the equilibrium and conceal the true extent of deficiency. Hypokalaemia may develop during nutritional support as potassium is taken into cells along with glucose.

Hypophosphataemia may develop if phosphate is not administered and may be associated with marked muscular weakness. Where prolonged starvation has been present, excessive nutritional repletion with large amounts of carbohydrate can lead to abrupt and profound hypophosphataemia, cardiac dysrhythmias and even death (refeeding syndrome). For this reason, nutritional support should be introduced gradually in profoundly malnourished patients, adequate amounts of phosphate supplied and serum electrolyte concentrations monitored carefully. Tetany can occur but is usually the result of hypomagnesaemia per se rather than hypocalcaemia. Excessive gastrointestinal losses of magnesium are usually responsible and are not uncommon in patients with high-output stomas or short bowel syndrome. Chronic diuretic therapy often contributes to a pre-existing deficiency. Magnesium depletion generally represents an indication for parenteral supplementation because the loss cannot be corrected adequately by enteral administration of the electrolyte.

Energy requirements and supply

Energy requirements are highly variable and difficult to predict, particularly in critically ill ventilated patients. Although sophisticated equipment has been devised to allow direct measurement of energy requirements by collecting and analysing respiratory gases (indirect calorimetry), measurements are difficult to perform and results have been shown to vary widely between individuals and even in the same individual at different times of day. Historically, critically ill patients have been given large amounts of energy, often in excess of requirements, and certainly far in excess of maximal rates of glucose utilisation. In some critically ill patients given large amounts of glucose-based total parenteral nutrition (TPN), this resulted in complications, particularly related to excessive lipid deposition within the liver.

Carbohydrate (glucose) supplies approximately 4.2 kcal of energy per gram, as does protein (amino acids). If the latter is used solely as the energy source, however, there is a 'conversion cost' of about 30% of total caloric value. Lipid is energy-dense and supplies approximately 9.1 kcal/g.

Very **few** patients require in excess of 2,500 non-protein kilocalories per day, and almost all patients can be fed adequately with 35 kcal/kg body weight. Since the use of glucose as a metabolic fuel leads to the production of more carbon dioxide than the oxidation of fat, large quantities of glucose administration may lead to critically increased respiratory workload in spontaneously breathing patients who have borderline or inadequate minute ventilation and elevated PCO_2. These potential difficulties can be avoided by using **lipid emulsions** in TPN and lipid-rich enteral feeding solutions. In critically ill patients, glucose intolerance may result in an inability to meet energy requirements if glucose is used as the principal energy source. The hyperglycaemia associated with insulin resistance may require the concomitant administration of large doses of insulin, which may increase the risk of fatty liver. Recent studies have also suggested that careful control of blood glucose concentrations in critically ill patients using insulin therapy may substantially improve prognosis and reduce infective complications. Common nutritional strategies incorporate **50%** of the energy requirements administered as lipid. Since the energy yield of lipid is higher than carbohydrate, the volume of feed required can be reduced

significantly. Concerns (controversial) about the effect of lipid emulsions on immune and pulmonary function in critically ill patients have led to recent caution over predominantly lipid-based regimens. In addition, some glucose is required in all feeding regimens to prevent ketosis. Glucose also helps to spare nitrogen by preventing the breakdown of muscle protein for gluconeogenesis (although its effect is reduced substantially in sepsis).

ENERGY REQUIREMENTS

- Energy requirements are difficult to estimate but in most cases can be assumed.
- Very few patients require in excess of 2500 non-protein kilocalories per day and almost all patients can be fed adequately with 25–35 kcal/kg body weight.
- Glucose (4 kcal/g) is often tolerated poorly in the critically ill.
- Excessive glucose administration causes fatty liver and disturbs liver function.
- Lipid (9 kcal/g) should provide around 50% of non-protein calories.

Protein requirements

The normal adult subject requires at least 50 g of protein each day. The biological value of individual proteins varies considerably depending upon the mixture of amino acids within them. The lack of an essential amino acid in a protein source or feeding solution greatly reduces the biological value. An essential amino acid is one that the body cannot synthesise from other amino acids by transamination in the liver. Some amino acids, *eg* glutamine, that are non-essential in health cannot be produced in quantities sufficient to meet the body's requirements in stress and are described as 'conditionally essential'. It is important to appreciate that, even in health, intake of protein in excess of requirements results in the excess being deaminated and the carbon skeleton used as an energy source (glucose). This is energetically inefficient. It is necessary to ensure that an appropriate amount of non-protein energy is supplied to avoid the unnecessary catabolism of protein. In the critically ill patient, this requires that about 100–120 kcal of non-protein energy is supplied for each gram of nitrogen.

Although the nitrogen content of individual amino acids varies, overall 6.25 g of protein provides

1 g of nitrogen. Most feed solutions are therefore designed with respect to their amino acid composition. It is thus more appropriate to talk in terms of nitrogen content rather than protein supplied. A maintenance diet should supply patients with approximately 0.15 g/kg/day of nitrogen. A depleted patient requires extra nitrogen and will need approximately 0.2 g/kg/day of nitrogen.

In the critically ill patient with SIRS or sepsis, the metabolic response and its associated exaggerated muscle protein catabolism result in elevated levels of circulating amino acids (along with elevated glucose and free fatty acids). Because the anabolic pathways are impaired by mechanisms that are understood incompletely, these plentiful substrates remain underutilised. Unused amino acids are ultimately deaminated in the liver, the carbon skeletons used for gluconeogenesis and the amine (nitrogen) group converted to urea. This results in increased urinary nitrogen losses. Additional sources of loss in such patients include drain fluid, wound exudate and even blood loss from arterial lines. In seriously ill patients, even with increased provision, continuing whole-body protein breakdown results in a continuing shortfall in the nitrogen economy.

A septic patient with these exaggerated losses may lose up to 0.3 g/kg/day of nitrogen. It is generally **not possible** to balance losses of nitrogen in these patients, but this does not mean that feeding should be discontinued. The most that can be hoped for is the attenuation of net negative nitrogen balance. Nutritional support has been shown to increase the rate of protein synthesis but does not affect the rate of protein catabolism, which continues unabated. Overall, the effect of feeding the critically ill is to halve net protein catabolism. Positive nitrogen balance (indicating repletion of visceral and muscle protein) is unlikely to be restored to septic patients unless the **underlying cause of sepsis is dealt with**.

PROTEIN/NITROGEN REQUIREMENTS IN SURGICAL PATIENTS

Healthy patient: about 0.15 g/kg/day of nitrogen.
Critically ill patient: about 0.2–0.3 g/kg/day of nitrogen.
Non-protein energy/protein ratio: 100–120 kcal/g N.
Intervention to deal with the underlying cause of sepsis/SIRS is the most important means by which nitrogen balance can be restored.

Trace elements and vitamins

Detailed knowledge of the exact requirements for trace elements, vitamins and minerals is beyond the scope of this chapter and is not required for the clinician to provide effective nutritional support for critically ill patients. Most commercially available feeding solutions will contain sufficient trace elements, vitamins and minerals to prevent the development of deficiencies. Certain deficiency states occur with sufficient frequency in surgical patients to merit comment.

Trace elements are found in micromolar concentrations (hence the name) in tissues. Zinc, copper, manganese, iodine, chromium, iron, cobalt, selenium and molybdenum have all been shown to be required (albeit in small amounts). Deficiency of some or all of these has been recognised in surgical patients and can usually be detected by combining clinical suspicion with laboratory assays.

Zinc deficiency is liable to occur when depleted patients are subjected to additional stress, such as major abdominal surgery or critical illness. In addition to depletion as a result of undernutrition, catabolic states are associated with exaggerated loss of zinc in the urine. Manifestations of zinc deficiency are especially likely when patients recover from critical illness, at a time when demand for zinc increases in association with synthesis of new protein. Zinc deficiency is manifest by apathy, depression, diarrhoea, skin rashes and alopecia. A total of 100 µmol of zinc each day is usually sufficient to prevent deficiency, although larger amounts of parenteral zinc may be required in cases where there is a large gastrointestinal loss, *eg* associated with diarrhoea.

Selenium is involved in antioxidant defence and is essential for the activity of glutathione peroxidase. Antioxidant defences play an important role in protecting tissues from damage associated with the generation of oxygen free radicals. This is particularly likely to arise in the critically ill. Selenium levels fall rapidly in acutely ill surgical patients and this may reflect consumption of selenium. More prolonged deficiency may give rise to cardiomyopathy, which may be irreversible. Daily administration of 0.4 µmol of selenium is usually sufficient to prevent deficiency.

Vitamins are organic molecules required to maintain normal cellular function. Commercially available diets, whether enteral or parenteral, include normal daily vitamin requirements. The effect of serious illness upon these requirements and the interaction between changes in requirements and the capacity of the patient to adequately assimilate vitamins presented either enterally or parenterally is not known. In the chronically debilitated alcoholic patient, thiamine deficiency still occurs surprisingly frequently. Vitamin C deficiency is difficult to assess but should be assumed if the clinical picture is suggestive. If in doubt, addition of supplements of standard vitamin preparations and trace elements is more likely to be beneficial than harmful.

NOVEL SUBSTRATES

Current provision of nutritional support to patients other than those with simple undernutrition must be regarded as suboptimal. Our present understanding of the factors that control and maintain the exaggerated breakdown of lean body tissue observed after major injury, and particularly in critical illness, is not sufficiently adequate to allow us to intervene effectively to reverse or prevent catabolism. Nutritional support should be regarded, at best, as an exercise in damage limitation. In recent years, interest has centred upon the use of a series of new (and expensive) nutrients in the hope that they may provide more effective nutritional support in critical illness. It is hoped that many of these nutrients will influence immune function and intermediary metabolism (see Table 11.4), but convincing clinical evidence of benefit is still awaited.

Table 11.4 *Novel substrates of possible immunological benefit*

Glutamine
Arginine
RNA
Branched-chain amino acids
Omega-3 fatty acids

Gastrointestinal failure

The concept of intestinal failure is useful: intestinal failure can be said to exist when the functioning intestinal mass of a patient is reduced below the minimal amount necessary for the adequate digestion and absorption of food. Like renal failure, intestinal failure is the end result of many different disease processes (see Tables 11.5 and 11.6). It is also a continuum ranging from temporary mild dysfunction to complete and irreversible failure needing chronic 'replacement therapy'. At one extreme, intestinal failure may be an acute reversible problem (*eg* small bowel obstruction) and at the other a chronic condition resulting from an irreversible loss of gut mass (*eg* mesenteric vascular occlusion). Renal failure can be diagnosed on the basis of simple laboratory tests, but intestinal failure is a clinical diagnosis based upon a history and examination, laboratory investigations and, in some cases, radiological investigations. Establishing a diagnosis of intestinal failure is important because attempts to provide enteral nutritional support alone are likely to be ineffective and early parenteral nutrition should be considered, possibly with referral to a specialised unit.

Table 11.5 *Underlying diseases associated with intestinal failure*

Crohn's disease
Pancreatitis
Peptic ulceration
Mesenteric vascular occlusion
Malignancy
Intestinal trauma (including surgical injury)
Diverticular disease
Radiation enteritis

Table 11.6 *Clinical problems associated with intestinal failure*

Enteric fistulation
Short bowel syndrome
Abdominal abscess
Motility disorders
Intractable diarrhoea
High-output stoma
Extensive parenchymatous small bowel disease

Parenteral nutrition is likely to be required in the patient with intestinal failure or in critically ill patients with combined gastrointestinal fluid losses in excess of 1 l/day. It has been traditionally held that, in critical illness, disturbed intestinal motility precludes enteral feeding. It is now clear that, in the majority of cases, ongoing ileus is confined to the stomach and colon and enteral nutritional support can be provided using nasojejunal or tube jejunostomy feeding techniques (see below).

INDICATIONS AND ROUTES FOR NUTRITIONAL SUPPORT

Nutritional support is indicated in any patient unable to take an adequate dietary intake for **more than three or four days**. If the gastrointestinal tract is working and access to it can be obtained safely, then enteral feeding should be initiated because it is cheaper and safer and has physiological advantages. The barrier function of the small intestine appears to decline rapidly if luminal nutrients are not provided, and this may increase the ability of bacteria and endotoxins to translocate across the intestinal wall, possibly contributing to the development of multiple organ failure. The mass and surface area (villous height) of the small bowel also decrease rapidly, which increases the risk of diarrhoea on resumption of feeds, which in turn may lead to feeding being withheld. Liver dysfunction, hyperglycaemia and septic complications (especially pulmonary) are significantly less common with enteral than parenteral nutrition.

The algorithm suggested by Hill (see Appendix) is proposed as a useful starting point for decision-making regarding the optimum route for nutritional support.

Enteral nutrition support may be achieved by the use of a naso-enteric tube (nasogastric, nasoduodenal, nasojejunal), or by tube enterostomy placed at the time of surgery, or as a separate surgical procedure, or percutaneously, with the aid of an endoscope.

> **BASIC RULES FOR ENTERAL NUTRITION**
> Enteral nutritional support should be considered when:
> - spontaneous oral intake is inadequate;
> - the proximal small intestine is intact and functional;
> - stimulation of secretory function does not clearly worsen the condition being treated (eg proximal small bowel fistula).

Supplementary enteral feeding

Supplementation of the diet with 'sip feeds' may be very useful when patients have a poor appetite but are able to drink. Current sip feeds typically provide 200 kcal and 2 g of nitrogen per 200 ml and are available in a variety of flavours. They may be useful in enabling patients to make the transition back to a full diet, and there is some evidence to suggest that they may reduce hospital stay and increase the speed of postoperative recovery. Their use, however, tends to replace rather than supplement food intake, and despite manufacturers' best efforts many patients still find them unpalatable. Chilling sip feeds and offering a range of flavours may help.

Nasogastric feeding

Feeding through a nasogastric tube is the easiest means of enteral feeding, but it is reliant on the adequacy of gastric emptying, which, as already indicated, is one of the last aspects of gut function to recover after an operation or major insult. High gastric residuals and gastric distension predispose to vomiting or the much more dangerous problem of regurgitation and aspiration. Any impairment of consciousness greatly increases this risk. Keeping the patient at least 15 degrees head up may reduce this risk significantly.

Judging when gastric emptying is adequate can be difficult. In the fed state, the stomach can produce up to 2,500 ml of secretions per day (in addition to receiving 1,500 ml of saliva each day). The normal gastric residual volume is between 50 and 100 ml, which represents the equilibrium between secretion and emptying plus absorption. Continuous passive drainage or suction through a conventional wide-bore nasogastric tube may lead to a large cumulative total over 24 hours even in the face of normal gastric emptying, because the gastric residual is replaced as quickly as it is removed. Pinning the bag up at shoulder height or spigotting the tube and aspirating at two-, four- or six-hour intervals will give a better indication of whether the stomach is emptying adequately. If volumes of 200 ml or less are returned, it will be easier to judge whether the volumes are increasing progressively, and the risks are relatively small. Most stresses and illnesses as well as many drugs increase gastric residual volume but may not necessarily lead to a degree of impaired emptying that would prevent feeding. Feeding can be commenced through a standard large-bore nasogastric drainage tube, but a fine-bore tube is better tolerated once the need for drainage is judged to have passed. Aspiration of gastric fluid through a fine-bore tube is much more difficult.

Nasojejunal or nasoduodenal feeding

Where gastric emptying remains a problem, a weighted tube should be used and guided into the proximal small intestine. Ideally, this can be placed at surgery, but other options include the use of fluoroscopy to advance the tube beyond the pylorus, endoscopic placement or the use of the 'Bengmark' tube, which has a coiled end and is propelled distally by peristalsis. In the patient with a reduced conscious level, radiological confirmation of the position of any feeding tube is mandatory because of the devastating consequences of instilling feeding solution into the lung.

Tube enterostomy

Where patients are undergoing laparotomy, consideration should be given to the insertion of a tube enterostomy as a planned part of their management. For example, tube jejunostomy should be considered in patients undergoing oesophagectomy, total gastrectomy or pancreaticoduodenectomy, or a laparotomy for abdominal trauma. Insertion of feeding tubes (as a separate procedure) should be considered when it is clear that enteral nutritional support is indicated and is going to be required for more than six weeks. Tube gastrostomy can be fashioned using one of two traditional techniques: the Stamm and Witzel techniques. Tube jejunostomy can also be accomplished using a catheter introduced over a fine needle, passed submucosally before entering the small bowel. In all cases, the bowel should be sutured to the abdominal wall deep to the site at which the catheter passes through the parieties. Minimal-access techniques can also be used to create tube enterostomies. Percutaneous endoscopic gastrostomy and transgastric jejunostomy are appropriate in the management of patients in whom laparotomy is not indicated but who need enteral nutritional support for a prolonged period. All of these techniques have significant complications, particularly small bowel obstruction due to tube migration and volvulus around the fixed insertion site, site infection or leakage of feed and peritonitis, due to separation of gut from the abdominal wall (see Tables 11.7 and 11.8).

Initiation of enteral feeding

There are a number of reasons why the gradual introduction of enteral nutrients is wise, but it is important to realise that efforts to establish feeding can be derailed by many things and one can easily

Table 11.7 *Indications for enteral nutrition*

Moderate-to-severe PEM with inadequate oral intake for more than three days
Dysphagia for all but clear fluids
Massive enterectomy (to encourage adaptation)
Distal enterocutaneous fistulae
After major injury (especially head injury) in patients in whom return to full oral intake will be prolonged
Prolonged recovery
Some patients with inflammatory bowel disease

Table 11.8 *Contraindications to enteral nutrition*

Complete small bowel obstruction
Inadequately treated shock states (may be associated with a risk of intestinal ischaemia)
Severe diarrhoea (low rate of feeding may be continued as it may improve absorptive surface)
Proximal small intestinal fistulae
Severe pancreatitis (unless fed distal to pancreas)

find that weeks have passed and adequate nutrition has still not been established satisfactorily. Common problems are cessation because of gastric residuals that are perceived to be too large, diarrhoea and dilution of feeds. Poor gastric emptying can often be overcome by the use of prokinetics such as metoclopramide.

For most patients, a standard, isocaloric (*ie* 1 kcal/ml) enteral formula is perfectly adequate. A useful regimen in patients with an otherwise normal gut is to start at 20 ml/h for six hours, then increase by 20 ml/h and repeat the process. If gastric tubes are used, aspiration to assess the gastric residual can be performed before each increment.

Table 11.9 *Complications of enteral feeding*

Related to intubation of the gastrointestinal (GI) tract
Fistulation
Wound infection
Peritonitis
Displacement and catheter migration (including small bowel obstruction)
Blockage of tube
Related to delivery of nutrient to the GI tract
Aspiration and hospital-acquired pneumonia (especially if feed is contaminated)
Feed intolerance
Diarrhoea

Dilution of feed is seldom required, as the intrinsic gut secretions ensure dilution of these small starting quantities. If there is reason to believe that absorptive capacity will be a problem (prolonged disuse leading to villous atrophy, significant small bowel resection), then the progression to full feeding (25–35 kcal/kg/day) may need to be much more gradual, otherwise diarrhoea will be inevitable.

DIARRHOEA

Diarrhoea can be a major problem in enterally fed patients (see Table 11.10). The commonest identifiable cause is concomitant administration of antibiotics, because of depopulation of the normal gut flora and direct irritant effects. If the latter can be stopped, diarrhoea will usually resolve rapidly. Other contributory factors include loss of absorptive surface because of villous atrophy or resection. The effect of the former can be minimised by striving to keep some enteral intake going all the time, or by reintroducing it a short time after surgery, even if it falls well short of meeting total nutritional needs. Glutamine is particularly important as a luminal nutrient for enterocytes, along with arginine, whereas the energy requirements of colonocytes are met principally from short-chain fatty acids derived from luminal fermentation of soluble fibre. Although feeds enriched with glutamine and fibre are available, it is unclear whether they lead to less diarrhoea than standard feeds. Diarrhoea is also more likely to occur when enteral nutrition is delivered via the stomach as opposed to the small intestine in patients with severe hypoalbuminaemia. The risk of diarrhoea can be minimised by introducing the feed gradually and by patiently increasing the rate. If diarrhoea does ensue, then a reduction to 20 ml/h is preferable to cessation in terms of limiting the overall duration of the problem, even though the volume of diarrhoea may be greater in the short term.

Clearly, it is important to rule out superinfection with *Clostridium difficile* or other bacterial dysenteries before treating with agents to slow gut transit. Once cleared, however, the use of loperamide, codeine or kaolin–pectin mixtures may be very helpful, especially after small bowel resection.

Parenteral nutrition

TPN can be defined as the intravenous provision of all nutrient requirements without the use of the gastrointestinal tract. This technique developed in the 1960s as a result of technological advances in both feeding solutions and intravenous catheters. Indications for TPN in surgical patients are shown in Table 11.11.

11.11 *Indications for TPN in surgical patients*

Obstruction of the gastrointestinal tract, eg patients with proximal small bowel obstruction that cannot be relieved immediately and who require preoperative feeding

Short bowel syndrome: patients with less than 300 cm of functional small intestine usually require at least temporary TPN. In many cases, adaptation will eventually permit enteral nutrition alone. Patients with less than 100 cm of small bowel generally require lifelong TPN

Proximal intestinal fistulae

Refractory inflammatory disease of the gastrointestinal tract

Inability to use the gastrointestinal tract for other reasons

Table 11.10 *Management of diarrhoea in the enterally fed patient*

Exclude infectious causes:
    Send stool for culture, including *Clostridium difficile* toxin
    Send feed for culture

Reduce load on gut:
    Consider jejunal rather than gastric feeding
    Reduce rate of delivery of feed (try 20 ml/h)
    In patients with short bowel, consider reducing gastric hypersecretion with omeprazole

Treat diarrhoea empirically:
    30 ml kaolin–pectin down tube every four hours
    Loperamide 2–4 mg twice daily

Other measures (unproven):
    Consider use of fibre- or glutamine-containing feeds
    Consider giving intravenous albumin if hypoalbuminaemia thought to be contributing to malabsorption

Short courses of parenteral nutrition can often be administered through dedicated fine-bore peripheral cannulae placed in the proximal cephalic vein. Alternatively, a fine-bore (22G) cannula can be inserted and replaced in a different vein every 24 hours. The chief limitation associated with the peripheral delivery of intravenous nutrition is the high incidence of thrombophlebitis. This can be reduced by ensuring that the hypertonic glucose content of the feed is minimised and by adding heparin and hydrocortisone to the feeding regimen.

Thrombophlebitis may also be reduced by promoting venodilation by applying a nitrate patch over the vein. Peripheral parenteral nutrition is safer than central venous feeding because the risks inherent in central venous cannulation are avoided and the consequences of catheter-related sepsis are generally less serious. The inability to easily deliver more than 3 l of fluid each day together with nutrition and the short half-life of peripheral venous cannulae (even dedicated fine-bore cannulae rarely last more than two weeks) makes the central venous route preferable for nutritional support, particularly in critically ill patients.

If possible, a **dedicated** line should be used for the administration of TPN. It should be inserted in the subclavian (lowest infection rate) or internal jugular vein and **tunnelled** to an infraclavicular position. Tunnelling reduces the rate of catheter infection. The tip of the line should be screened into the distal superior vena cava because this promotes maximal mixing of the feeding solutions with venous blood, reducing the risk of catheter-associated thrombosis. Intravenous feeding via the femoral vein should be avoided if possible because the incidence of line infection and catheter-related complications is higher. The exit site should be protected carefully with an occlusive dressing, and full aseptic technique should be used when dressings are changed or the line is handled. The potential severity of line sepsis should not be underestimated, and a **high degree of suspicion** must be maintained in any patient with central access of any type who develops signs of infection or deterioration without a clear explanation. Most units performing TPN regard line sepsis rates above 6% as unacceptable. When a multilumen catheter has to be used, one channel should be preserved solely for TPN and the above precautions observed as far as possible.

CHOICE OF SOLUTION FOR PARENTERAL NUTRITION

Nutritional assessment should allow for estimation of the likely energy and nitrogen requirements of the patient. Most hospital pharmacies have ready-compounded 'big bags' containing different volumes of TPN solutions, of varying composition. They provide a range of calorie/nitrogen ratios, as outlined above, and the non-protein energy source is composed of either glucose alone or a lipid/glucose combination. The metabolic abnormalities encountered in sick surgical patients generally necessitate the use of lipid

as a 50% energy source, so that hyperglycaemia can be avoided. The volume of feed is tailored to the patient's fluid requirements. In the preparation unit, the lipid is usually added last, to maximise stability of the lipid emulsion. Adding subsequent compounds can easily lead to 'cracking' of the lipid emulsion and is to be avoided. Divalent cations (such as Ca^{2+} and Mg^{2+}) are a particular problem.

TPN should be administered via an accurate, electronically controlled infusion pump. Stable patients can often be fed on a cyclical, usually nocturnal basis. This allows the patient to mobilise during the day. In the critically ill patient, the large volumes of fluid required and/or the need to avoid rapid swings in the state of hydration usually make continuous feeding over 24 hours mandatory.

Table 11.12 Complications associated with the provision of TPN

Catheter-related
　Mechanical: blockage, central vein thrombosis, migration, fracture, dislodgement
　Infective: exit site infection, line sepsis, infective endocarditis
Metabolic
　Hyperglycaemia: too much glucose infused (occasionally seen in severe sepsis)
　Deranged liver function: cause unclear but may relate to biliary stasis and excessive calorie administration, with fat deposition in liver
　Hypoglycaemia: too rapid cessation of glucose infusion
　Hypertriglyceridaemia: too much lipid infusion
　Hyperchloraemic acidosis: too much chloride in nutrient solution

MONITORING THE PATIENT DURING NUTRITIONAL SUPPORT

Institution of nutritional support should follow the same systematic plan as other forms of management.

There is seldom, if ever, a need for immediate nutritional intervention. Attention to the ABCs and underlying causes assumes greater importance. Although patients with sepsis certainly require nutritional support, the limited efficacy of nutritional support in the presence of active sepsis makes **management of sepsis** the most important step in the nutritional management of the critically ill patient.

As discussed earlier, no simple laboratory tests

can measure the benefit or otherwise of nutritional support. Albumin and other visceral proteins are markers of systemic disease activity and SIRS rather than the state of nutritional wellbeing. Creatinine, urea and electrolyte estimations should be performed daily to assist in adjusting the constituents of the feed. Full blood count, serum concentrations of calcium and magnesium, and liver function tests need less frequent (usually weekly) testing in the stable patient (see Table 11.13).

Table 11.13 *Haematological and biochemical investigations in the assessment and monitoring of nutritional status in stable patients*

Daily (if stable)
   Full blood count
   Glucose (may need feeding and fasting samples)
   Urea, creatinine and serum electrolytes
Weekly (if stable)
   Magnesium, calcium, phosphate
   Chloride
   Albumin
   Bilirubin
   Transaminases
   Gamma-glutamyl transpeptidase
   Alkaline phosphatase
   Prothrombin time
Twice-monthly (if stable)
   Vitamin B_{12} and folate
   Iron and iron-binding capacity
   Copper, zinc, selenium
   Prealbumin, transferrin

In long-term patients, estimations of zinc, iron studies, vitamin B_{12}, red blood cell folate and visceral proteins such as fibrinogen are useful at intervals of weeks to months (see Table 11.13).

It is exceedingly difficult to assess and monitor the nutritional status of the critically ill patient since major weight changes reflect sequestration of water rather than nutritional repletion or depletion. Changes in muscle mass may be difficult to evaluate clinically in a grossly oedematous patient, and changes in plasma proteins frequently reflect the existence of sepsis rather than nutritional depletion. The most appropriate route of feeding and amount of nutrition provided can be planned at this stage, as described above, and reassessment of the patient's needs can be undertaken as sepsis improves.

PROPHYLACTIC FEEDING

The place of 'prophylactic' perioperative feeding has been controversial for many years. While there is no doubt that malnourished patients have more operative morbidity and a higher perioperative mortality rate than normally nourished patients, there are surprisingly few scientific data to support the use of perioperative feeding. In particular, perioperative TPN has been shown to increase the operative morbidity (particularly from sepsis), especially in patients with only mild-to-moderate malnutrition. It is reasonable to suggest that markedly malnourished patients (> 10% weight loss) should, if possible, be offered preoperative nutritional support. Where possible (see above), this should be provided by the enteral route. There would appear to be little value in a period of feeding of less than seven to ten days' duration. Patients with active infection will not benefit from preoperative feeding, and the cause of sepsis should be dealt with by radiological or surgical means at the earliest opportunity.

PREOPERATIVE NUTRITIONAL SUPPORT
- There is no clear scientific evidence of benefit from preoperative nutritional support.
- Drainage of sepsis takes precedence over attempts to provide preoperative nutritional support.
- Short courses of preoperative nutritional support (less than 7 days) are entirely ineffective.

SUMMARY

Nutritional support of the critically ill patient is a frequently neglected but integral part of the delivery of surgical care. Just as the support of the cardiovascular and respiratory systems of critically ill patients is based upon an understanding of the altered physiology associated with disease, so nutritional intervention is based upon an understanding of the metabolic processes in the critically ill. The ultimate goals of nutritional support in the surgical patient are to ensure that the patient is optimally prepared for the stress of a surgical procedure and that recovery, even in the face of complications, is associated with minimal depletion of body stores.

- Think about nutrition.
- Assess status and requirements.
- Select route and amount.
- Check that delivery has been successful.

Fluid and electrolyte management   **12**

Objectives

This chapter will help you to:

- Be better able to manage complex fluid balance in critically ill patients.
- Understand the physiology of water and electrolyte balance and distribution as applied to the critically ill.

- Be aware of the common deficiencies and excesses and their causes and management.

INTRODUCTION

Assessing fluid balance and prescribing appropriate fluid is an important daily task for surgeons. As the registrar, it will be often be your responsibility to ensure that this is carried out safely and accurately. In many surgical patients, the process becomes potentially complex because of multiple sources of fluid loss and several types of fluid input. However, with a logical approach and a clear understanding of a few basics, even complex cases can be dealt with. Conversely, poor prescribing remains a common cause of avoidable morbidity.

FLUID COMPARTMENTS AND CONTROL OF VOLUME

The total body water volume (approx. 45 l) is distributed through the intracellular and extravascular compartments in a ratio of 2 : 1. The total volume of water is controlled by both central osmoreceptors and volume receptors that affect thirst and the release of antidiuretic hormone (ADH). It is important to remember that activation of the volume receptors will release ADH even in the face of hyponatraemia and a low plasma osmolality. This is the rule of the **primacy of volume** for ADH release.

Extracellular fluid volume is maintained by the presence of sodium and its accompanying anions,

which are largely excluded from the intracellular compartment by the action of the sodium/potassium pump. Volume and pressure receptors control sodium retention and excretion, and the body has a very rapid response to a fall in central volume or renal perfusion by reducing renal sodium excretion to extremely low levels. In critical illness and after surgery, the obligatory extracellular volume required to maintain adequate venous return to the heart rises due to the loss of salt water and protein into sites of tissue damage, obstructed bowel, serous body cavities and the relaxation of the peripheral vascular bed. In some situations, *eg* sepsis, the amount of sequestered fluid may be prodigious. The volume sequestered may cause a search for other causes of circulatory failure and thus delay adequate fluid resuscitation. Later, the sequestered fluid may cause problems of circulatory overload during recovery as it is remobilised.

- Intracellular volume is maintained by the solute contained within the cells, the most important single cation being potassium.
- Assessment of fluid and electrolyte status requires both clinical and biochemical examination.
- The extracellular compartment is easier to assess clinically as increased salt and water manifests as oedema, while salt and water depletion is manifest by effects on the circulation.

- Intracellular volume is extremely difficult to assess clinically, and biochemical measures are used as a proxy.

BIOCHEMICAL ASSESSMENT

Normal basal requirements for sodium are 80–100 mmol/24 h, but this can vary a lot with surgical illness. Conversely, drug solutions can contain significant amounts of sodium. Care must also be taken to ensure that a false value for sodium is not obtained by venepuncture from a limb with a running fluid infusion or if there is frank lipaemia (hypertriglyceridaemia due to inherited disease or secondary to intralipid administration).

Hyponatraemia

Often, the concentration of sodium ions in the plasma gives a much clearer idea of the relative water state of the body than of the sodium or salt status. **Clinical assessment** of the patient is essential in addition to having a biochemical measurement, as a patient with hyponatraemia of, for example, 125 mmol/l may be sodium-depleted (hypovolaemic), sodium-replete or sodium-overloaded (oedematous due to cardiac, renal or hepatic disease), dependent upon the relative quantity of water to salt in the extracellular space. Table 12.1 lists some of the types and causes of hyponatraemia.

The management of hyponatraemia may be by rapid sodium chloride infusion, water restriction or diuretic plus water restriction, dependent upon clinical assessment. It must be remembered that water cannot be excreted by the kidney in the presence of extracellular fluid (ECF) depletion (see above) and that the syndrome of inappropriate ADH secretion

(SIADH) can be diagnosed only once the patient has been shown to be in sodium balance.

Correction of hyponatraemia should be achieved at a rate similar to that at which it developed. In chronic states, the rapid achievement of a normal value may precipitate massive water shifts, with severe consequences, particularly in the brain. The use of hypertonic saline is seldom necessary, and in the presence of normal renal function water overload can be cleared by the administration of diuretic and 0.9% sodium chloride to replace the fluid excreted by the kidney.

Hypernatraemia

This can be caused by abnormal intake or administration of hypertonic fluid, *eg* 8.4% sodium bicarbonate, but it is more commonly due to abnormal water loss (diabetes insipidus or mellitus, osmotic diuretics, fever or high environmental temperature) in a situation where intake of water is impaired. Correction is with water administered by the **gut** for preference or by intravenous 5% dextrose. Occasionally, 0.45% saline may be required to avoid an excessive sugar load, particularly in patients with diabetes mellitus.

Hypokalaemia

The usual requirement for potassium is 60–100 mmol/day. The level of potassium in the blood is a very poor reflection of the total body potassium content, as the plasma contains only 1% of the body total. The maintenance of the cellular transmembrane gradient is important for normal neural and muscle function, and the rate of change of the extracellular potassium concentration is more important than the absolute value. Maximum urinary conser-

Table 12.1 *Hyponatraemia: types and causes*

Urinary sodium	ECF volume		
	Low (NaCl −−−, H_2O −)	Normal/slightly raised (NaCl normal, H_2O +)	High (NaCl +, H_2O +++)
High (>20 mmol/l)	Diuretics (excessive)	Glucocorticoid deficiency	Renal failure
	Salt-losing renal disease	Hypothyroidism	
	Mineralocorticoid deficiency	Syndrome of inappropriate secretion of ADH	
Low (<20 mmol/l)	Extrarenal loss:		Cirrhosis
	1 Outwith body		Cardiac failure
	2 Sequestration		Nephrotic syndrome

vation of potassium takes between one and two weeks to achieve, and even with normal renal function urinary levels (5–10 mmol/day) never fall to the minimal levels found for sodium in salt depletion (0–1 mmol/day). Hypokalaemia is usually the result of loss of potassium from the body via the kidney or bowel (diuretics, tubular disease, diarrhoea or laxatives) (see Table 12.2). Acute changes in plasma potassium may occur as potassium moves into cells during the correction of an acidosis, secondary to the acute release of catecholamines (cerebral bleed or trauma), administration of salbutamol or upon refeeding with the start of anabolic activity. The level should be kept above 3.5 mmol/l by stopping any avoidable losses and the administration of potassium.

Table 12.2 *Common causes of hypokalaemia in surgical practice*

Renal losses
Intestinal losses
Medical losses: no potassium in the drip!

Hyperkalaemia

A rapidly rising plasma potassium level is a medical emergency and will result in respiratory muscle weakness and cardiac arrest from which it is extremely difficult to be resuscitated.

The primary route of potassium excretion is via the kidney in the distal nephron under the influence of aldosterone. Renal failure, hypoadrenalism, distal nephron disease (*eg* chronic obstructive nephropathy) or drugs that affect the renin–aldosterone system (*eg* ACE inhibitors) will all impair the excretion of potassium. Where there is a sudden movement of potassium out of cells due to trauma, drugs (suxamethonium), ischaemic/hypoxic damage or a sudden rise in hydrogen ion concentration, patients with impaired renal excretion will be particularly vulnerable. *A classic example is the hypovolaemic patient with a metabolic acidosis plus respiratory compensation who has anaesthesia induced with suxamethonium: the patient is then underventilated, with a consequent sudden fall in pH, and suffers a cardiac arrest shortly after induction.*

There is no absolute level above which the signs and symptoms appear, and effects are related to the rate of rise as much as to the plasma concentration.

A chronic potassium level of 6.0 mmol/l will be tolerated well but may be fatal if the result of a rapid change from 4 mmol/l. Levels this high require rapid specific treatment (see Chapter 8) plus reversal of the primary condition and removal of any precipitant drugs if possible.

Calcium

The calcium level in the plasma is normally kept within a narrow range under the influence of parathyroid hormone, 1,25-dihydroxy-vitamin D_3 and renal function. The active component is the ionised fraction that is unbound to albumin. Total levels have to be regarded in relation to the albumin level, or the ionised fraction has to be measured directly.

HYPERCALCAEMIA

Severe hypercalcaemia will affect neural tissue and damage renal tubular function. In the critically ill patient, this will rarely be due to hyperparathyroidism or vitamin D intoxication; more often, it is due to paraneoplastic hypercalcaemia associated with solid neoplasms such as carcinoma of the breast or multiple myeloma. Hypercalcaemia diminishes the kidney's ability to retain salt, and the resultant hypovolaemia reduces the ability of the kidney to excrete calcium. A variety of dysrhythmias may occur. Establishing a saline diuresis will normally help reduce the level. If this fails, the administration of a bisphosphonate intravenously will reduce the level of calcium. Effective treatment of the primary cause will also bring the level back to normal. The development of hypercalcaemia in association with recurrence of a solid tumour is usually an indication of a poor prognosis.

HYPOCALCAEMIA

Apparent severe hypocalcaemia may be found in the critically ill patient if the total plasma level is measured without reference to the albumin level. An absolute hypocalcaemia level is seen in acute pancreatitis, vitamin D deficiency, acute rhabdomyolysis and following thyroid surgery when all parathyroid tissue has also been removed. Treatment is by the administration of calcium, treatment of the primary condition and, in post-parathyroidectomy syndrome or vitamin

D deficiency, administration of activated vitamin D analogues. In those situations of critical illness with intact parathyroid function, aggressive administration of calcium should be limited to situations where there is **clinical** evidence of hypocalcaemia rather than attempting to achieve a given value.

Magnesium

Magnesium is the most important intracellular cation after potassium. Magnesium is essential for the normal functioning of nerve and muscle. Depletion causes confusion and seizures and is associated with a range of dysrhythmias, while excess causes muscle paralysis and central nervous depression. Significant hypermagnesaemia is almost always secondary to iatrogenic administration in the presence of impaired renal function, *eg* as magnesium sulphate for eclampsia. Hypomagnesaemia is secondary to poor diet plus losses from the bowel or kidney and, rarely, congenital renal tubular disorders. Long-term loop diuretic therapy, chronic malabsorption or diarrhoea, and alcohol abuse are the commonest causes. In the critically ill, hypomagnesaemia is common in the early recovery period of severe insults such as faecal peritonitis. As with potassium, plasma levels reflect total body magnesium poorly, but a plasma level below 0.6 mmol/l associated with a condition likely to cause magnesium deficiency or the presence of symptoms should precipitate supplementation. This is best done intravenously in the acute stage to avoid the purgative effects of magnesium salts. The plasma level should not exceed 1.5 mmol/l. Critically ill patients with dysrhythmias should have magnesium levels checked, as treatment with magnesium contributes to the control of several dysrhythmic states.

Phosphate

Phosphate is present in any protein-containing food and is absorbed from the gut. The kidney excretes phosphate under the influence of parathyroid hormone. High levels will be seen in renal impairment or following massive muscle or bowel necrosis. In the short term, this is usually not a major problem unless large quantities of calcium are administered. Hypophosphataemia is commonly seen in the critically ill, usually following the correction of the primary problem. As cell function is restored, phosphate is taken back into cells with potassium and magnesium. When the phosphate level falls below 0.6 mmol/l, there are effects that can be measured regarding **respiratory** and other skeletal muscle function plus effects upon the functioning of the immune system. Replacement will come with refeeding, but with levels below 0.6 mmol/l intravenous supplementation will be required given slowly over 24 hours.

Trace metals

There are many trace metals that are essential to normal cellular function and the healing process, *eg* zinc and selenium. In situations where there is prolonged dependence upon parenteral feeding or prolonged gut dysfunction, consideration must be given to the measurement and necessary supplementation of their intake.

CLINICAL ASSESSMENT

The patient should be assessed fully according to the CCrISP system. Take particular note of sources of fluid intake and loss. Relate these to the patient's underlying condition, operative treatment and timing, comorbid diseases and drugs. Along with clinical examination, the fluid balance chart is the principal mechanism of assessment, but accuracy of fluid balance charts is variable and with experience one learns which wards[1] charts can be relied upon. There is no one formula that can be applied to all situations, and regular frequent clinical assessment of the patient will be required to adjust the content and volumes of fluid replacement assisted by biochemical measurement of the blood, urine and other fluid being lost from the body, *eg* fistula fluid. Particularly with chronic overload, daily weighing of the patient, when feasible, can be of assistance and complements the fluid balance chart.

APPROACH TO THE PRESCRIPTION OF FLUID AND ELECTROLYTES

This section should be read in conjunction with Provision of requirements in Chapter 11.

In the critically ill, fluid replacement will be guided by the clinical situation, which is constantly changing. Requirements will be dependent upon many factors, including:

- body weight (determines basal requirements);
- estimated existing fluid and electrolyte excess or deficit;
- continuing insensible loss of water dependent upon fever;
- continuing loss from gastrointestinal tract;
- continuing loss from renal tract; and
- other effects of recent surgery, such as fluid redistribution (third space) and loss from open wounds.

Fluid isotonic for sodium will be required to maintain adequate extracellular volume.

Water orally or dextrose will be needed to maintain intracellular volume and provide sufficient volume in which to excrete the renal load of solute waste.

The total volume of clear intravenous fluids prescribed will need to be reduced depending on the volume being given by other routes or forms (drugs, oral intake, nutrition, blood, etc).

Electrolyte deficiencies will need to be corrected as well as basal needs being met.

Replacing abnormal losses

As a general rule, abnormal losses should be replaced with a fluid having the same composition as that which is being lost, and in a similar volume. However, matching the fluid exactly is not always necessary, as the kidneys compensate efficiently under many circumstances.

Losses can be divided into those that consist more or less of ECF or its equivalent, and those that are mainly or purely water. Clearly, some conditions have elements of both (see Table 12.3).

Table 12.3 *Abnormal fluid losses*

Losses that approximate ECF	Losses that are principally water
Blood loss	Fever
Vomiting	Increased respiratory rate
Diarrhoea	Prolonged water deprivation
Gut fistulae	Diabetes insipidus
Postoperative 'third-space' sequestration	
SIRS, *eg* sepsis, burns, pancreatitis	
Diabetes mellitus (hyperglycaemia)	

When there is loss of an ECF-equivalent fluid, there is a decrease in the total ECF volume, including the plasma volume. This deficit should be replaced promptly to restore perfusion to cells and vital organs. Abnormal losses of water with or without electrolytes (particularly sodium and potassium) will result not only in a reduction in plasma volume but also in a marked change in intracellular fluid volume and the concentrations of important ions across cell membranes. Restoration of the plasma volume always takes precedence and should be accomplished with a balanced salt solution (see below).

Restoration of the water deficit and other electrolyte deficits can then be addressed. This should be accomplished gradually so that rapid shifts of water across membranes, especially the blood–brain barrier, are avoided. It takes much longer for electrolytes to equilibrate between some compartments than others, and the resulting osmotic gradient can lead to fatal cerebral oedema or other complications if therapy is too hasty. Aim to correct these over 48–72 hours.

REPLACING EXTRACELLULAR FLUID LOSS

Central to the replacement of ECF deficits (blood volume, interstitial volume) is the use of a balanced salt solution. This term refers to a crystalloid solution that is isotonic (and remains so) and has constituents that are similar to the ECF (physiological saline or 0.9% sodium chloride, lactated Ringer's, also known as Hartmann's solution). When a balanced salt solution is given, it will distribute itself throughout the extracellular compartment (approximately 14 l) over several minutes. Only about one-third of the volume given will remain in the vascular space. Understanding this phenomenon will prevent undertreatment of blood volume deficits when using balanced salt solutions. Reduced intravascular volume is usually accompanied by an interstitial fluid deficit. Redistribution of balanced salt solution into the interstitial space is therefore usually desirable.

In a situation where the volumes required are large, maintenance water and electrolytes often get forgotten. This seldom matters in the first 24 hours or so, because the volume shifts are so large and the kidney can usually sort out what it wants to keep or excrete. However, as time goes on, maintenance water needs to be thought about, otherwise the patient will become hypernatraemic and hyper-osmolar.

VOMITING, DIARRHOEA AND INTESTINAL FISTULA LOSSES

These gastrointestinal conditions cause losses of fluid that resemble ECF, although typically of a lower osmolality (*ie* more water is lost relative to sodium). The result is blood volume depletion, dehydration and large electrolyte losses. If water has been taken only orally to try to compensate, hyponatraemia may be present, but if serum sodium is normal or even high, then the possibility of a significant sodium deficit must not be overlooked. In some conditions (*eg* vomiting from complete upper small bowel obstruction, diarrhoea due to cholera), the volumes lost can be huge and rapidly life-threatening.

Potassium depletion is universal, and may be severe with marked diarrhoea. Metabolic acidosis may mask the extent of total body potassium deficit by causing potassium to move from within cells to the extracellular compartment in exchange for extracellular hydrogen ions.

Additionally, vomiting or nasogastric drainage leads to loss of hydrogen (H^+) and chloride (Cl^-) ions from the stomach. This can produce a marked meta-bolic alkalosis, but despite this it is rare that H^+ needs to be given intravenously. Adequate chloride replacement in the form of 0.9% saline will usually correct the deficit, as endogenously produced acid (H^+) will be retained by the kidney.

By using fluid balance charts and clinical assess-ment logically to keep total volume and key ions, particularly sodium and potassium, in balance, you can achieve success in the great majority of cases. However, there is no single formula for success and patients change continually, so reassess.

Case history 12.1

A 58-year-old 70-kg man, otherwise fit except for longstanding atrial fibrillation controlled with digoxin, underwent a cystectomy for bladder cancer three days ago. An ileal urostomy was constructed, necessitating a small bowel anastomosis. Presently, he is on the HDU, he is apyrexial and his chest is clear (respiratory rate 16/min), but his abdomen is rather distended. Although his urine output is rather low, he seems reasonably well perfused. The monitor shows atrial fibrillation at a rate of 118/min. It is Saturday and you are on call. The HDU nurse has asked you to sort out the patient's fluid balance for the weekend. Review the fluid bal-ance chart below and prescribe his intravenous fluid. His consultant wished him to stop antibiotics after 72 hours.

What further information do you require?

What would you prescribe, and how?

Are blood tests necessary today?

When should you review further?

Answer to case history 12.1

This is clearly a complex case who is not yet clini-cally stable. In addition to making your own clinical assessment, you should review the fluid charts from the previous day or two to look for patterns and for accumulating losses or excesses. Look at the opera-tion note for any specific postoperative orders. Urinary anastomoses may leak for a few days, so urine appears through the drain as well as the catheter and/or urostomy. Ileus can be prolonged and nutritional support may be needed, but again this is not pressing at 72 hours postoperative. You clearly need to review yesterday's biochemistry results (sodium 138, potassium 3.1, urea 5.2) and repeat these today. Summate the data above and include insensible loss – about 750 ml is probably reasonable here, but revise the factors that influ-ence this.

The patient's needs are probably about 3,500 ml – the water requirement (5% dextrose 2,000 ml) will be unchanged – the excess volume should be crystalloid (1,500 ml). His antibiotics will be stopped but his PCA

Intake summary Last 24 hours	CVP line 0.9% saline (975 ml)	Peripheral line (R) Dextrose 5% (1,800 ml)	Peripheral line (L) Antibiotics (600 ml), PCA (125 ml	Oral Sips (120 ml)
Losses summary Last 24 hours	Nasogastric tube 1450 ml	Pelvic drain 720 ml	Urostomy 640 ml	Bowels Nil, no flatus

will continue. You will need to give at least some of the fluid via the CVP line to keep it open. He is hypokalaemic and you should aim to give 80 mmol of potassium over the next 24 hours; you may modify this when you review with the blood results later. This need is the more pressing because of his atrial fibrillation and digoxin therapy. If potassium replacement and digoxin fail to control the rate, then the magnesium level should be ascertained.

It is obviously inappropriate to prescribe for the whole weekend just now. Some losses, such as the nasogastric loss, may increase or decrease, and clinical and biochemical reassessment is needed. Plan to review with your team at the end of today and again at 8am tomorrow.

SUMMARY

- Patient size and age.
- Abnormal ongoing losses, pre-existing deficits or excesses, fluid shifts.
- Renal and cardiovascular function.
- Look at the fluid balance chart for the last 24 hours:
  - are all fluids given or lost included?
  - do the volumes seem right from other available information?
- Check previous charts for insidious changes.
- Serum electrolyte values (note limitations).
- Use urine electrolytes, weight and plasma osmolality when needed.

Pain management 13

Objectives

This chapter will help you to:

- Understand the effects and risks of inadequate analgesia.
- Learn to function as a member of a multidisciplinary team providing analgesia in the critically ill patient.
- Understand your role in the management of acute pain throughout the continuum of surgical care, from the general ward through to the HDU/ICU.
- Acquire the knowledge to decide on the appropriate method of analgesia and the skills necessary for your role in its deployment.
- Be aware of the systemic effects of analgesia and the complications of analgesic techniques.

INTRODUCTION

Nociception is the term given to the reception of a noxious or unpleasant stimulus and its conversion into an impulse transmitted up a sensory nerve. Pain refers to the perception of that sensation in the central nervous system and the recognition of it as unpleasant. Suffering is the emotional response that makes one miserable and is associated with the severity of the pain and its duration.

Society relies on doctors to provide relief of pain and suffering. It is important for all doctors to have a fundamental understanding of pain, including how it is generated and perceived. As members of the surgical team, you will look after patients presenting with primarily painful conditions and will encounter pain produced by surgical operations and interventions.

Safe and effective management of acute pain is an integral part of surgical practice. Although the physical status of the patient, the degree of trauma and the available techniques may be very different, the principles involved are similar whether the patient is recovering from major surgery on a general ward or being managed in the HDU/ICU.

Good-quality analgesia is essential for humanitarian reasons alone, but there are also compelling medical reasons for its provision. Inadequately controlled pain increases sympathetic outflow, leading to an increase in heart rate, vasoconstriction and increased oxygen demand, particularly in the myocardium, where it may contribute to infarction. It may impair lung function; abdominal and thoracic procedures almost always lead to impaired respiratory function because the pain induced by movement inhibits coughing and diaphragmatic function, leading to the atelectasis/pneumonia sequence.

Pain is not always bad, however. Pressure ischaemia resulting from resting on a body part for a prolonged period produces pain, causing the person to move off the affected area, thereby avoiding damage from pressure necrosis. Pain causes people to rest and protect already injured areas, preventing further damage and allowing healing.

PRINCIPLES OF ACUTE PAIN MANAGEMENT

The realistic aim of pain relief is not to totally abolish pain in the postoperative period but to ensure that patients are **comfortable** and have **return of function** with a more rapid recovery and rehabilitation. There are several important principles relevant to the provision of good-quality pain relief.

Prevention

The single most important step we can take in alleviating pain is to prevent the factors that produce it. Avoiding tension during surgical closure may help, as may preventing drains or tubes from pulling on sutures, or relieving urinary retention.

The use of drugs to prevent the development of pain is **more effective** than the treatment of existing established pain. This is the concept of pre-emptive analgesia. In practical terms, this means that local anaesthetic drugs or other analgesic agents should be given before rather than after surgical trauma.

Recognition of new problems

,It is critical that trainee surgeons are able to recognise when a patient's pain has altered to a point where an alternative explanation is required. Any patient who has escalating analgesic requirements needs to be assessed with a high degree of suspicion. **Ischaemia** is a common trap, as are bleeding, anastomotic leakage and compartment syndrome. 'Breakthrough pain' in a patient who previously had effective analgesia should be treated as a surgical complication until proven otherwise.

Managing expectations

The two most powerful forces in play during pain management are the expectations of the patient and those of the healthcare staff. If either believes that the patient will be in severe pain, then the outcome will tend towards that result; if both believe the converse, then the outcome is likely to be fewer complaints and more rapid mobilisation.

Preoperatively, patients should be told to expect significant pain. They should also be told that pain can be controlled by various means, and that they will not be allowed to suffer. If the patient is distressed by their pain, or if pain is inhibiting their breathing or their ability to cough, then a change in technique will be required.

Surgical considerations

Upper abdominal incisions are associated with considerably more pain, more pulmonary disturbance and more difficulty effecting adequate analgesia than lower or transverse abdominal incisions. The choice of site and type of incision are therefore important in the sick patient who has limited respiratory reserve. Postoperative pain management will be aided by the use of local anaesthetic infiltration at the time of surgery or by specific local and regional anaesthetic techniques. Epidural infusion analgesia is the most commonly used of these techniques; other examples include caudal blocks for perineal surgery, intercostal blocks for cholecystectomy, and ilioinguinal blocks for lower abdominal incisions.

THE ROLE OF THE SURGICAL TRAINEE IN THE MULTIDISCIPLINARY ACUTE PAIN TEAM

The provision of postoperative pain relief has always been hindered by confusion about whose responsibility it is to perform this function. Traditionally, postoperative analgesia has been prescribed by the anaesthetist, administered by the ward nurses and supervised by a junior surgical trainee. The Joint College Working Party Report on Postoperative Pain recommended that each major hospital should have a multidisciplinary acute pain team consisting of surgeons, anaesthetists, nursing staff and pharmacists. With increasingly sophisticated methods of analgesia being used, it is vitally important that the surgical trainee liaises with the other members of the team and is aware of protocols and guidelines relating to acute pain management in the hospital.

> **Practice point**
> As the clinician likely to be contacted first in the case of a surgical patient becoming critically ill, the surgical trainee must establish:
>
> - whether poor pain relief is contributing to the patient's lack of progress; and
> - whether the method of analgesia is contributing to the patient's deterioration.

PATIENT ASSESSMENT AND MANAGEMENT

Immediate management

In the critically ill patient in pain, patient assessment is vital. It should follow the same system of assessment as in any other circumstance.

AIRWAY

Start at the beginning by checking that the patient has a patent airway. Oversedation secondary to opioid drugs may be associated with episodic airway obstruction. This is particularly marked in patients who are elderly, are obese, have a history of obstructive sleep apnoea (OSA) or who have had surgery to the head or neck. It may be exacerbated by the administration of other sedative drugs, such as benzodiazepines.

Practice point

Episodes of airway obstruction and resultant hypoxaemia often persist for two to three nights after major surgery. Supplemental oxygen should be continued for **at least 72 hours** in high-risk patients recovering from major surgery who receive any form of opioid analgesia (including PCA and by the epidural route).

BREATHING

Check the respiratory rate and the pattern and depth of breathing. Is your patient's respiratory function impaired by inadequate analgesia? Can the patient cough and expectorate properly to avoid problems later? The rational use of opioid analgesia has always been limited by the fear of drug-induced respiratory depression. A much more common problem is the patient slowly slipping into respiratory failure due to poorly controlled pain that is inhibiting movement and the ability to cough.

Practice point

- Respiratory rate is an unreliable indicator of opiate-induced respiratory depression. Sedation levels are a more sensitive indicator of impending opioid overdosage.
- Severe hypoxaemia may occur in the presence of normal respiratory rates.
- Poorly relieved pain, particularly in upper abdominal surgery, is a major cause of failure to cough, sputum retention and hypoxaemia.

In the assessment of the critically ill patient in pain, it is therefore essential to assess the adequacy and depth of the respiratory pattern as well as respiratory rate, and to check the patient's ability to cough. Investigations including arterial blood gas analysis and continuous pulse oximetry can be useful adjuncts to clinical findings when assessing a patient's respiratory adequacy (see Case history 13.1).

Case history 13.1

You review a 52-year-old man on the morning of the second postoperative day following a suture repair of an incisional hernia, which had occurred in an old upper midline scar. Initial assessment shows the patient to be well built (95 kg), a little drowsy but adequately rousable. His breathing is rapid (24/min) and shallow, and he cannot breathe deeply enough for you to hear his breath sounds well. He is sweaty and tachycardic (110/min) but normotensive' and well perfused. A pulse oximeter showed an SaO_2 of 88% initially; this has risen to 92% with mask oxygen at 6 l/min. He has a past history of smoking and mild chronic bronchitis. Review of his charts shows that four-hourly morphine 10 mg has been given for analgesia.

You think that he is hypoxic, largely because of poor analgesia.

You increase the flow rate of oxygen to 12 l/min and ask for it to be humidified. The patient's conscious level improves and he affirms that he is in pain from his wound. It is 90 minutes since his last analgesia, so you give a further 10 mg intramuscular morphine. After 20 minutes, the patient is more comfortable. Auscultation now reveals reasonable air entry but some expiratory wheeze. Salbutamol (2.5 mg in 5 ml) is given by nebuliser.

Blood gases (on 12 l oxygen) show:
PO_2 150 mmHg (20 kPa), FiO_2 0.6
PCO_2 53 mmHg (7 kPa)
pH 7.29
BE 0.4 mmol/l
HCO_3^- 28 mmol/l.

There is a mild respiratory acidosis and hypercapnia and an acceptable oxygen concentration.

You arrange for review by the on-call physiotherapist and for a chest radiograph. After discussion with the pain team, arrangements are made for PCA to be established, and you prescribe regular paracetamol six-hourly and rectal diclofenac 50 mg eight-hourly (having previously noted that he has normal renal function).

You review the patient at lunchtime. Repeat

blood gases one hour after physiotherapy show marked improvement. With continuous pulse oximetry, the oxygen flow is reduced steadily to 6 l/min. The patient is comfortable, breathing well and able to cough at will.

Learning points

- Poor analgesia is common and has profound effects on respiratory and other vital organ function – four-hourly as-required opioids are often inadequate.
- Analgesic techniques are generally better at preventing pain than at rescuing a patient from marked discomfort with associated complications.
- Review the effect of interventions – reassess your patient.
- A multidisciplinary approach can be very useful in pain management.

CIRCULATION

A persistent tachycardia or hypertension caused by inadequate analgesia may potentiate the development of myocardial ischaemia, particularly in the patient who is already hypoxaemic. A common clinical problem is the differential diagnosis of hypotension occurring in the patient receiving epidural analgesia following major surgery (see later). This is often attributed to the epidural infusion and the relative hypovolaemia secondary to vasodilation. Patients with sympathetic blockade are very sensitive to inadequate volume replacement, and care must be taken in these patients to replace fluid losses immediately. This requires meticulous attention to the maintenance of accurate fluid balance charts, measurements of losses from surgical drains and a high index of suspicion for concealed losses.

> **Practice point**
> Persistent hypotension in this group of patients may be due to postoperative surgical bleeding, and this should always be borne in mind.

DISABILITY

It is important to assess whether the method of analgesia is contributing to the patient's clinical deterioration. Particular attention should be paid to the patient's level of consciousness, as decreasing conscious level is an early indicator of opioid toxicity.

Full patient assessment

CHART REVIEW

If pain relief is felt to be contributing to the patient's deterioration, then the drug charts should be reviewed with the following questions in mind:

- Is effective analgesia prescribed?
- Is effective analgesia being given?
- Is the treatment appropriate for this patient?

The recorded pain and sedation scores should be reviewed and the scores repeated (see below).

HISTORY AND SYSTEMIC EXAMINATION

The contribution of pain to the patient's general condition should be ascertained during your full patient assessment.

Behavioural observations

Assessment of pain by hospital staff is usually based on the patient's outward response, or 'pain behaviour'. Verbal complaints, facial expression, restriction of mobility and changes in heart rate and blood pressure are used intuitively to build an impression of how much pain a patient is suffering. While these are often good predictors of pain, it is important to realise that, in some individuals, such assessments may be quite wrong and we may significantly under- or overestimate the level of suffering.

Severity scoring systems

The effectiveness of assessment of analgesia will be increased vastly if simple reproducible pain scoring systems are used. These systems emphasise restoration of function by assessing pain scores during movement and when coughing (see below). Pain scores should be recorded when the patient is taking deep breaths, is coughing and on movement, otherwise the score may be falsely low.

PAIN SCORING SYSTEMS

Verbal rating scale – is your pain:

0 = absent?

1 = mild?

2 = discomforting?

3 = distressing?

4 = excruciating?

Numerical rating scale – which number describes your pain?:

0	5	10
No pain		Worst imaginable

Visual analogue scale

{————————————————}

No pain   Worst imaginable

Functional assessment:

• Can you move?

• Can you cough?

Practice point

Pain scoring in the patient recovering from major surgery should be as done as routinely as measurement of blood pressure or respiratory rate.

INVESTIGATIONS

Investigations assessing respiratory function are used frequently when assessing the adequacy of analgesia. Serial arterial blood gas analysis and CXRs are often used to demonstrate trends in respiratory capacity, and sputum cultures are essential when planning antibiotic therapy.

DECIDE AND PLAN

If pain relief is adequate and the patient is improving, then continue and review. If pain relief is inadequate, then determine why:

• Is it due to failure of the method of analgesia?
• Is it due to incorrect implementation of the method chosen?
• Is it due to the development of a surgical complication?

Pain relief is not the only important factor in the postoperative period, but it should be considered as an integral part of the patient's total care. In certain situations, the method of analgesia may determine whether the patient has a smooth postoperative course or becomes critically ill. In a patient who has pre-existing chest disease, for example, the analgesic technique chosen when an upper abdominal incision is planned may determine whether a period of postoperative ventilation on the ICU is required.

TECHNIQUES AVAILABLE FOR THE MANAGEMENT OF ACUTE PAIN

It is important for all those involved in the delivery of pain services to understand the range of techniques available. At one end of this spectrum is the administration of single analgesic agents, often given orally, to a patient in mild discomfort. As the intensity of pain increases, there is a need for an increased response from those providing the pain relief. In some cases, increased analgesic requirements may be met by increasing the dose or potency of the drugs used. Other situations will demand the use of more sophisticated regimens. Combinations of methods and agents may be needed (multimodal therapy). Alternatively, effective analgesia may require the use of sophisticated techniques, such as PCA or epidural infusion analgesia (EIA).

It may be helpful to think of the increasing level of intervention required with increasing pain in terms of an 'analgesic ladder' (see Fig. 13.1). As a patient's pain intensity escalates, so does the level of support needed. When the situation improves, and the intensity of the pain decreases, analgesic requirements will also decrease, and a technique from lower down the ladder can be used.

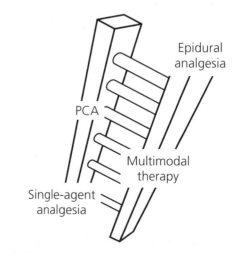

Figure 13.1 *Analgesic ladder*

> **Practice point**
>
> The use of a technique from higher up the analgesic ladder does not necessarily mean stopping more simple techniques; epidural analgesia can be often be supplemented effectively by the use of regular paracetamol or NSAIDs.

> **Practice point**
>
> Opioids must be administered by only one route at a time: respiratory and other toxic effects from epidural opioids will be potentiated if oral, intramuscular or intravenous opioids are given concurrently. Such toxicity is potentially fatal.

Single-agent analgesia

Except in minor pain or discomfort, it is unusual for optimal analgesia to be obtained from a single agent or technique. If single-agent analgesia is used, it will be more effective if drugs are prescribed and administered **regularly** rather than on an as-required basis. All analgesic drugs can be given as single agents but are usually more effective when given as part of a **balanced multimodal therapy regimen**.

Multimodal therapy

It is often difficult to produce safe, effective analgesia with a single group of drugs. Better results with fewer side effects are achieved if combinations of drugs affecting different parts of the pain pathway are used. Such balanced analgesia (multimodal therapy) usually consists of a combination of local anaesthetics, opioids, NSAIDs and paracetamol.

Analgesic agents

PARACETAMOL

This is a very useful drug, which has a high therapeutic index and very few side effects in normal dosage. It is toxic in overdose because it depletes the glutathione reserve of the liver and then damages hepatocytes. Paracetamol should be given regularly, and can be administered by the oral, rectal or, more recently, intravenous (as the prodrug pro-paraceta-

mol) routes. It should form the basis of most in-hospital pain regimens.

NON-STEROIDAL ANTI-INFLAMMATORY DRUGS

NSAIDs are used increasingly as part of balanced analgesia as adjuncts to opioid analgesia in an attempt to increase efficacy and reduce opioid side effects. Different preparations are available for dosing by sublingual, oral, rectal and parenteral routes. NSAIDs are unlikely to be chosen for the management of pain relief in the critically ill patient, due to their effects on haemostasis and renal function.

> **Practice point**
>
> NSAIDs are often contraindicated in critically ill patients due to their potentially disastrous effects on renal function and gastric mucosa.

The cyclo-oxygenase 2 (COX-2) inhibitors are a newer subgroup of NSAIDs enjoying great commercial success. However, they are substantially more expensive than standard NSAIDs and accumulating evidence suggests that gastrointestinal side effects may not be substantially different and that efficacy is no greater. The true place of these agents remains to be defined.

OPIOIDS

Opioids remain the gold standard of analgesia when a potent agent is required for severe pain. Morphine is the commonest and cheapest agent available. The principles discussed below apply to all opioids, as do the toxic effects.

Codeine phosphate

Codeine is an opioid with weak analgesic properties. In randomised, controlled trials, it has an efficacy equal to paracetamol in adequate dose. However, it is profoundly constipating and may produce substantial nausea, which limits its usefulness. It is often used in combination preparations, presented with paracetamol.

Tramadol

This drug has been popular in Germany for many years and recently enjoyed a surge in popularity in many other countries. It has many opioid-like properties but without the same extent of respiratory depression or the tendency to produce dependence. It does, however, have a marked emetic effect in many patients.

Oral morphine

Although the bioavailability of morphine is quite low by the oral route, adequate effect can easily be achieved with dose titration. It carries with it all the usual potential side effects of opioids. Patients with short-term needs or in transition to oral medication are best managed with morphine elixir. For chronic pain, a slow-release tablet form may be most appropriate. Other opioids are also available orally or as slow-release transcutaneous patches (fentanyl).

Intravenous opioids: bolus doses

Adequate analgesia is achieved most rapidly by an intravenous bolus dose, or repeated doses if the desired effect is not achieved with the initial dose. Often, boluses of 5 mg are given initially, followed by further increments of 1–2 mg until satisfactory analgesia is achieved. This may require surprisingly large doses – 20–30 mg is commonly needed in an average-sized patient to produce good pain relief.

Once analgesia is achieved, intravenous dosing is commonly maintained by self-administration of further doses (*ie* PCA; see below).

Intravenous opioid infusions

Although opioid infusions can be very effective, respiratory and other side effects are common, and they should be used only in an ICU setting. Intravenous opioid infusions are therefore beyond the scope of the CCrISP course and will not be considered further.

Intramuscular opioids

The intermittent, as-required prescription of intramuscular opioid analgesia was once the traditional form of postoperative pain relief. However, the use of four-hourly intramuscular injections has been shown repeatedly to be ineffective in a high proportion of patients recovering from abdominal surgery, and this technique has now been superseded by more effective methods of analgesia.

Opioid side effects

The limiting factor for use in the conscious postoperative patient is the emergence of side effects in a dose-dependent progression. All opioids exhibit similar effects, although the profiles of different agents may differ in the detail.

Respiratory depression: all opioids reduce the sensitivity of the respiratory centre in the brainstem in a dose-dependent manner. Even in therapeutic doses, the partial pressure of carbon dioxide (PCO_2) will show an elevation from the normal value (5.3 kPa = 40 mmHg). A high normal PCO_2 of up to 6.5 kPa should be considered an expected consequence of using such drugs (as should constricted pupils) and is not a reason to stop using them. Both respiratory rate and tidal volume are affected by opioids. Respiratory rate is easier to measure at the bedside, and it is extremely unlikely that dangerous respiratory depression will occur without a fall in rate below the normal range (12/min in adults).

Sedation: a decreasing level of consciousness carries with it the risk of loss of protective reflexes, especially those associated with protection of the airway (cough, gag and the ability to recognise imminent regurgitation). As unconsciousness deepens, airway occlusion may occur.

> **Practice point**
> A low respiratory rate will usually improve by stopping administration of opioids. If the respiratory rate falls below 8/min, or if the patient becomes hypoxic, or if the patient is at risk from a decreased level of consciousness, then small doses of the opioid antagonist naloxone may be indicated (100 µg repeated until the desired effect is achieved). Be aware that naloxone may produce dysphoria, hypertension, tachycardia and the sudden and unwelcome return of severe pain if it is not titrated carefully.
>
> Remember that the half-life for an intravenous dose of naloxone is short – approximately 15–20 minutes – and symptoms may reappear.

Nausea and vomiting: this is a distressing and common side effect. It is dose-related and is potentiated by movement and when gastric emptying is already impaired. It is caused both by direct stimulation of the chemoreceptor trigger zone (CTZ) in the medulla and by gastric distension. Unfortunately, there is little evidence that the common practice of prophylactically administering antiemetics such as metoclopramide, prochlorperazine or cyclizine has any effect on the incidence of this complication.

Patient-controlled analgesia

Although PCA has been available for 30 years, it has only become used widely in the past 10 years. The technique is based on the concept of the patient self-administering a bolus dose (usually 1 mg) of morphine intravenously, after which the PCA machine will allow no further demands for a predetermined period – the 'patient lockout' time. During this lockout period, which is usually set at five minutes, the patient is unable to receive further doses. After the lockout time has elapsed, the patient is able to repeat the dose of analgesic drug if they are still in pain. In this way, the patient titrates their own level of analgesia, increasing demands when requirements are high (eg during physiotherapy) and reducing them when needs are lower or if they experience side effects.

PCA is well accepted by patients and nursing staff, gaining high levels of patient satisfaction and providing good-quality analgesia. The efficacy and safety of the technique depends upon the factors shown in Table 13.1.

Table 13.1 Checklist for PCA

Does the patient understand PCA?	√
Do the staff understand PCA?	√
Is the patient the only person pressing the button*?	√
Is the pain responsive to opioids? Check pain score	√
Is the patient receiving any other opioid or sedative drug?	×
Is the patient receiving a background infusion?	×
Is the patient being monitored appropriately?	√

*See nurse-controlled analgesia below

The major advantage of PCA is that it gives the patient control of their analgesia and greatly reduces the fear of unrelieved pain. It is also intrinsically safe; if the patient becomes sedated, they will administer no further drug, blood levels will fall and they will recover consciousness.

Sleep disturbance is a major problem with use of PCA. The requirement for regular dosing may prevent the patient having adequate periods of undisturbed sleep. Often, the pain is severe by the time the patient reawakens and takes some time to bring under control.

PCA is unsuitable for patients who are confused or who are unable to press the demand button for physical reasons. In these circumstances, nurse-controlled analgesia is an alternative.

Epidural analgesia

The most effective way of producing profound analgesia is to block afferent pain pathways by the use of epidurally administered local anaesthetic drugs.

INSERTION OF THE EPIDURAL CATHETER

This procedure is usually performed by the anaesthetist responsible at the time of surgery. Both lumbar and thoracic approaches are used, the latter commonly being used to provide analgesia for both thoracic and abdominal surgery.

> **Practice point**
> Many anaesthetists will not insert an epidural catheter if the patient has received even one dose of anticoagulant prophylaxis, so it is worth consulting with the anaesthetist if preoperative heparin or low-molecular-weight heparin is being considered.

ADMINISTRATION OF EPIDURAL DRUGS

The anaesthetist will have checked the position of the epidural catheter (ensured that it is in the epidural space, excluded accidental subdural or subarachnoid placement) by giving a test dose of local anaesthetic, and will have established an infusion before the patient leaves the theatre suite. The infusion will usually be a mixture of a dilute concentration of local anaesthetic (bupivacaine 0.1–0.125%) with small amounts of added opioid (commonly fentanyl 2–4 μg/ml). Combinations of drugs are administered epidurally for similar reasons to combinations administered by other routes, ie better analgesia with fewer side effects.

The aim is to get good pain relief with minimal sympathetic effects and no motor block. Infusion rates of 8–15 ml/h are commonly used. A functioning epidural gives outstanding pain control.

TROUBLESHOOTING EPIDURALS

The two most common problems are breakthrough pain and hypotension. Close co-operation between the surgical team and the acute pain service, along with clear management protocols, is essential.

Breakthrough pain

This may be due to a problem with the epidural or the development of a new surgical problem. The patient should be assessed fully on each occasion and a new complication ruled out. Help should be sought from the pain team if it is apparent that the epidural is not functioning. An increase in the infusion rate (often preceded by a bolus or top-up dose) may be required, or the catheter may require repositioning.

Hypotension

Hypotension is a relatively common problem with epidural infusions, particularly in younger patients and in patients with higher-level blocks. If hypotension is caused by the epidural, it is usually due to sympathetic block and consequent vasodilation. As there are many other common causes of hypotension in the postoperative patient, the epidural must not be assumed to be responsible until other potential causes have been excluded. As always, when assessing the hypotensive patient with an epidural, use the CCrISP system of assessment (the ABCs) to avoid missing other causes (*eg* hypovolaemia, bleeding, MI).

Once it has been established that epidural-induced vasodilation is the cause of the hypotension, and once any hypovolaemia has been corrected, the pain team may decide to manage the problem by introduction of vasoconstrictors. This is beyond the scope of this manual, but agents used may include dopamine, noradrenaline and metaraminol. It is not usually necessary to stop the epidural infusion to treat hypotension, although this may be required in the short term if the hypotension is profound. If in doubt, ask your anaesthetic colleagues.

Case history 13.2

Eight hours after an uncomplicated right total knee replacement, you are asked to review a 59-year-old woman with ischaemic heart disease who has gradually become hypotensive (blood pressure 80/40 mmHg).

You assess the patient and find her alert, comfortable and with acceptable perfusion. Continuous epidural analgesia is in progress, using a mixture of fentanyl and bupivacaine in standard dosage. There has been no chest pain, dysrhythmia or hypoxia (lowest SaO_2 95%). Total volume in the drains is 750 ml, which the specialist nurse relates as 'average'. The wound is not soaked and the leg is not swollen. The patient has received saline at 150 ml/h since returning from theatre. The epidural appears to be working well; the block is infra-umbilical and the patient can move her toes.

You conclude that the patient is hypovolaemic but cannot decide whether postoperative blood loss or vasodilation from the epidural is predominant. In either event, a fluid challenge is needed, so you give 500 ml colloid over one hour. During this time, a full blood count shows Hb 11.0 g/dl.

Peripheral perfusion improves but blood pressure fails to respond. There are no signs of ongoing bleeding or of excessive epidural blockade or narcotisation (which can occur occasionally). An ECG shows no acute change. Given the history of ischaemic heart disease, you are reluctant to give a further fluid challenge without CVP monitoring. CVP proves to be +6 cmH_2O. You increase this to +10 with a further 500 ml of colloid over another hour, but the blood pressure rises to only 85/45 mmHg. Urine output in the last hour was 30 ml. You feel that this blood pressure is too low given the cardiac history and discuss matters further with the anaesthetic service. They concur and supervise the setting up of an infusion of dopamine, according to local policy. One hour later, with CVP maintained at +9, blood pressure is 105/65 mmHg and urine output has been 60 ml.

Learning points

- Hypotension associated with epidural analgesia is common: sympathetic blockade, perioperative bleeding and loss of fluid into tissues or through insensible losses can all contribute, and investigations are needed to establish the cause.
- Postoperative bleeding must be actively considered and dealt with.
- The need for treatment of hypotension due to the epidural alone depends on the pressure, comorbidity (especially cardiac or peripheral vascular) and the effect on end organs (urine output).
- All patients should be adequately filled with intravenous fluid, monitored by CVP and moved to the HDU as necessary.

- When the epidural is discontinued, the extra fluid administered will re-enter the circulation and can occasionally cause congestive cardiac failure in susceptible patients.

Other local/regional techniques

There are numerous other techniques based on the use of local anaesthetic agents, which may be encountered in specific circumstances. These range from simple intraoperative infiltration of the wound to nerve blocks, plexus blocks, intrapleural infusions and so on. All have their proponents and specific indications, but all work on the principle of blocking generation or conduction of the noxious stimulus to prevent it being perceived as pain.

CHRONIC PAIN

This is beyond the scope of this text, except to note that poor management of acute surgical pain may be one factor in the production of chronic pain and chronic analgesic dependence. Paradoxically, the latter is produced more often by inadequate use of analgesics rather than overuse, as is commonly believed.

WHERE SHOULD SUCH PATIENTS BE NURSED?

For many reasons, including the provision of adequate postoperative pain relief, all patients recovering from major surgery should be nursed in an area with a high ratio of nursing staff to patients. Any ward designated for the care of patients recovering from major surgery should have enough trained nurses and doctors to care for patients requiring PCA or epidural analgesia subject to the following provisions:

- The establishment of an acute pain service with named consultants responsible for the provision of postoperative pain relief.

- Rapid 24-hour availability of designated doctors and a resuscitation team.
- A system for monitoring patients on a regular basis, including pain scores, respiratory rate and sedation scores.
- Protocols and an education programme for all staff for the detection and management of major complications.
- Availability of continuous monitoring or transfer to an HDU or ICU for high-risk cases.

It is the responsibility of the acute pain service or a designated consultant to organise services such that the level of care and monitoring is appropriate for the clinical condition of the patients and the techniques of pain relief employed. Provision of adequate analgesia is often difficult and complex in the sick surgical patient: consideration should be given to transferring such patients to a higher level of care.

SUMMARY

- You are an essential member of the acute pain team, often being the first person called to a pain-related problem.
- When assessing the patient in pain, use the CCrISP system of assessment.
- Poor pain relief threatens the critically ill patient.
- Pain relief should provide comfort and restoration of function; analgesia should be assessed using reproducible pain scores and the ability of the patient to cough effectively.
- Multimodal therapy can dramatically improve pain relief and reduce side effects: remember the concept of the analgesic ladder.
- PCA and epidural analgesia are very effective techniques, but patients need careful monitoring and regular reassessment to prevent problems.
- *Be in regular contact with the acute pain team and your anaesthetic colleagues.*

Sedation **14**

Objectives

This chapter will help you to:

- Understand how acute confusional states may present in the critically ill.

- Be aware of management principles.
- Understand the limitations of drug therapy.

ACUTE CONFUSIONAL STATES

Confusional states are common during medical or surgical illness, particularly in the elderly, and are often worse at night. They are manifest by restlessness, a clouding of consciousness, loss of contact between the patient and the surroundings, inattention, disorientation in time, place and person, recent memory loss and agitation. There are often associated sleep disturbances, errors of perception, hallucinations and marked emotional lability. The safe and effective management of a ward patient with an acute confusional state is one of the most challenging problems facing the hospital doctor. The main aim of management should be to **identify and treat the cause**, although commonly none can be found. Treatment of the confusional state is often required before its cause can be sought and in order to allow specific therapy (*eg* **oxygen therapy**) to begin. Table 14.1 lists some of the causes of acute confusional states.

General management

Often, the most important aspect of treatment is keeping the patient oriented with the surroundings. Clocks, calendars, personal effects, rooms with windows and regular scheduled sleep periods will facilitate this, but the presence of a suitably trained person to observe and support the patient is essential. Interaction with the patient should be empathetic; attempts to reason with the patient are

Table 14.1 *Causes of acute confusional states*

Stress:
> Physical, eg hostile environment, invasive procedures, fatigue, disorientation
> Psychological, eg fear, anxiety, pain, discomfort, abnormal sleep patterns

Systemic disease:
> SIRS, respiratory failure, cardiac failure, renal failure, hepatic failure, pneumonia, urinary tract infection, hypoglycaemia, thyrotoxicosis, myxoedema, electrolyte (Na^+, K^+, Ca^{2+}) or fluid disturbances, acute porphyria, thiamine deficiency, alcohol withdrawal

Intracerebral disorders:
> Cerebrovascular accident, postictal state, head injury, haematoma, meningitis, encephalitis, abscess, tumour

Drugs:
> Tranquillisers, hypnotics, anticholinergics, opioids, tricyclic antidepressants, dopamine agonists, diuretics, digoxin, beta-blockers, steroids, NSAIDs

---

unlikely to be of benefit. In general, a quiet and calm environment should be encouraged. The use of bedside rails may add to patient safety.

Often, it may also be necessary to use sedative drugs. However, it should be remembered that **no** sedative agent or sedative technique is entirely safe. A full knowledge of the effects of common sedative agents is mandatory. Careful titration of sedative agents with monitoring of patient response will be the most successful and safe method of treatment. Treatment of the acutely confused patient is best undertaken in an HDU.

Assessment

After ensuring that the patient's airway, breathing and circulation are stable, the initial assessment of the confused or agitated patient is directed towards identification of the underlying cause (see below). Hypoxia and shock are common causes of confusion or agitation. Look actively for these and administer oxygen liberally, at least initially. Treat any underlying cause appropriately.

ASSESSMENT OF THE CONFUSED/AGITATED PATIENT

1 Ensure that the airway, breathing and circulatory status, etc, are stable.
2 Review the patient's case notes.
3 Take a full clinical history if possible.
4 Take note of the observations of ward staff caring for the patient.
5 Undertake a thorough clinical examination.
6 Investigate as necessary: haemoglobin, urea and electrolytes, blood sugar, serum calcium, arterial blood gas analysis, liver function tests, full sepsis screen, lumbar puncture, CT scan, EEG.

If pharmacological sedation appears necessary, then the patient's baseline level of consciousness should be assessed and documented on a sedation flowsheet. Once sedative drugs have been administered, regular re-evaluations of conscious level are mandatory. Assessment is best undertaken using an established sedation score, such as the Ramsay score (see Table 14.2). Using this scale, sedation should be **titrated** to produce a level between 2 and 4.

Table 14.2 *Ramsay sedation score*

Level of sedation	Patient response
1	Anxious and agitated or restless or both
2	Co-operative, oriented and tranquil
3	Quiet; responds to verbal commands
4	Asleep; brisk response to forehead tap or loud verbal stimulus
5	Asleep; sluggish response to forehead tap or loud verbal stimulus
6	Unresponsive

Modified from Ramsay MAE *et al. BMJ* 1974; **ii**: 656–9

Other monitoring during sedation should include **continuing, regular** assessments of:

- rate, depth and pattern of breathing,
- heart rate, and
- blood pressure.

Although the use of a pulse oximeter to measure peripheral oxygen saturation may be a useful adjunct to assessment, it should be remembered that, when a patient is receiving supplementary oxygen, life-threatening hypercapnia may occur despite normal SaO_2 levels.

DRUGS USED IN SEDATION

Drugs used to modify mood and behaviour are termed psychotropic agents. In general, they can be categorised into hypnotics/anxiolytic sedatives (*eg* benzodiazepines, trichloroethanol derivatives) and antipsychotic drugs (*eg* phenothiazines, butyrophenones). In acute emergencies, these drugs are best administered intravenously in small aliquots titrated to the desired effect. The elderly, the very ill, and patients with hepatic or renal dysfunction may be very sensitive to even small doses of sedative drugs. Alternatively, the intramuscular route should be used if intravenous access is impossible. In less acute situations, the oral route is preferred.

Benzodiazepines

These act by augmenting the action of gamma-aminobutyric acid (GABA) at receptors in the central nervous system. GABA is an inhibitory transmitter that opens chloride channels in the neuronal membrane, thereby reducing neuronal excitability. Benzodiazepines are well absorbed orally, but they can also be administered via the intravenous and intramuscular routes. They are metabolised in the liver, some to pharmacologically active metabolites. The half-life of different benzodiazepines varies considerably, with that of diazepam being relatively long compared with that of midazolam. Generally, when administered alone in clinical doses, benzodiazepines do not cause significant respiratory depression, but in conjunction with opiates they have a synergistic depressant effect on the respiratory centre.

EXAMPLES

Diazepam:

- oral 2 mg three times daily
- i.v. 2.5–10 mg
- i.m. 2.5–10 mg.

Midazolam i.v. 2.5–10 mg.

Trichloroethanol derivatives

Both chloral hydrate and triclofos are oral agents that are metabolised rapidly in the liver to the sedative trichloroethanol.

> **EXAMPLES**
> Chloral hydrate oral 500 mg–2 g.
> Triclofos oral 500 mg–2 g.

Phenothiazines

These drugs act by blocking many different neurotransmitter receptors, including those stimulated by dopamine, catecholamines, histamine, acetylcholine and 5-hydroxytryptamine (5-HT). They produce apathy and reduced initiative but possess unwanted effects, including postural hypotension, obstructive jaundice, autonomic effects, hypothermia and extrapyramidal motor disturbances. In very rare circumstances, they are responsible for the development of the neuroleptic malignant syndrome (hyperthermia, muscular rigidity, tachycardia and blood pressure lability). Many phenothiazines are absorbed erratically after oral administration. Additionally, there is a variable relationship between plasma levels and clinical effect. Intramuscular doses of phenothiazines are lower than oral doses because of the absence of first-pass metabolism.

> **EXAMPLES**
> Chlorpromazine:
> - oral 25–50 mg three times daily, increasing to 300 mg daily (use about one-third of these doses in the elderly)
> - i.m. 25–50 mg three times daily.

Butyrophenones

Like the phenothiazines, these drugs act by blocking many different neurotransmitter receptors, including dopamine, alpha-adrenergic, histamine, muscarinic and 5-HT receptors. Similarly, they may cause hypotension, extrapyramidal motor disturbances and the neuroleptic malignant syndrome. Haloperidol is particularly useful in the agitated, delirious patient and causes little respiratory depression.

> **EXAMPLE**
> Haloperidol:
> - oral 1.5–3 mg three or four times daily (max. 15 mg daily) (use about one-half of these doses in the elderly)
> - i.m. 2–30 mg three or four times daily
> - i.v. 1–5 mg.

Chlormethiazole

Chlormethiazole is related structurally to vitamin B_1 (thiamine). It is used particularly for the treatment of alcohol withdrawal. The intravenous form (0.8% solution) contains only 32 mmol/l Na^+, so clinically significant hyponatraemia is a potential side effect in long-term or high-dose use. The oral dose is one to two capsules or 250–500 mg as a syrup. For the treatment of alcohol withdrawal, the intravenous infusion can be administered at about 3–7.5 ml/min until light sleep is induced (*ie* Ramsay sedation score 4). Once this is achieved, a maintenance infusion of 0.5–1 ml/min may be administered, but sedation score and respiratory function must be assessed regularly.

Side effects of sedative drugs

Careful attention should be paid to the side effects of sedative drugs. Those common to most sedative agents are listed in Table 14.3.

Table 14.3 *General side effects of sedatives*

Depressed level of consciousness
Respiratory depression
Depression of cardiovascular system
Loss of airway tone leading to airway obstruction
Masking of other features of illness/deterioration
Reduced peripheral motor tone
Confusion
Immobility: skin pressure necrosis, rhabdomyolysis, venous stasis (DVT), dehydration, malnutrition

Treatment of overdosage

In the event that a patient develops coma or other more severe side effects of sedation, the following should be undertaken:

- Provide a patent airway using posture and an oropharyngeal or nasopharyngeal airway.
- Place the patient in the recovery position.
- Give high-concentration oxygen (*eg* facemask 15 l/min).
- Provide patient with ventilatory support using a self-inflating bag.
- Call urgently for anaesthetic or ICU support.
- Administer a suitable antagonist drug, *eg* flumazenil for benzodiazepine sedation.

ALCOHOL WITHDRAWAL

Symptoms and signs of withdrawal usually start within 24 hours of the last intake of alcohol. Initially, symptoms and signs include shaking, sweating, anxiety, agitation and confusion, but they can progress to hypertension, tachypnoea, hallucinations and seizure activity. If medication can be given orally, chlordiazepoxide (60–80 mg reducing by 10 mg daily over one week) is of particular benefit, as it reduces anxiety, tremor and agitation and prevents seizures and delirium tremens. If the oral route cannot be used, an intravenous infusion of chlormethiazole can be administered. Patients should also receive intravenous or intramuscular injections of vitamins B and C. Seizures should be treated using conventional anticonvulsants.

SUMMARY

- Treat the cause rather than simply the symptoms and signs of confusional state.
- Place patient in a quiet, calm environment.
- Provide experienced personnel to monitor the patient.
- Remember that sedation may be required in order that the cause can be identified or treatment begun.
- Use sedative drugs in small doses, titrated to the required effect.
- Regularly monitor the level of sedation using a sedation score and assessments of vital signs.
- Be aware of the potential side effects of sedatives, particularly airway obstruction and respiratory depression.
- Know how to treat airway obstruction and respiratory depression.
- If there are difficulties, call for help from the ICU as early as possible.

Objectives

This chapter will help you to:

- Understand the importance of a systematic approach, which includes initial assessment and resuscitation, secondary survey, continuing re-evaluation and monitoring, in-depth investigation and initiation of definitive care.
- Understand the importance of a continuum of care for the injured patient, often by a multidisciplinary team in which responsibility is **actively** shared.

- Know how to assess priorities during all phases of management.
- Appreciate the importance of frequent and **repeated** systematic assessments aimed at early detection of deterioration and previously unrecognised injuries.
- Know when to consider surgical intervention.
- Understand when to institute higher levels of care and when and how to transfer a patient safely.

BACKGROUND

In the western world, trauma is the principal cause of death between the ages of one and 40 years. In the UK, injured patients occupy more hospital beds than patients with cancer and heart disease combined. Approximately 10,000 people die each year as a result of accidents, almost 4,000 of these on the roads. Road traffic accidents account for 60,000 hospital admissions a year and industrial trauma a further 6,000. For every death from trauma, there are two people with permanent disabilities.

In England and Wales, a study of 1,000 consecutive trauma deaths showed that, in two-thirds of patients who died in hospital from thoracic or abdominal injuries, death could have been prevented by prompt and effective surgical intervention. In short, hospital doctors performing initial assessment missed life-threatening lesions in the abdomen and chest or failed to understand the significance of such injuries.

When death is plotted as a function of time after injury, there are three peaks in the resulting graph. The first peak represents those patients who die immediately or very soon after injury, usually at the site or in transit to the emergency department. These deaths are usually caused by laceration to the brain or spinal cord, heart or major blood vessels. With the exception of occasional deaths from airway obstruction, such deaths are rarely preventable.

The second peak represents people who die within the first few hours of injury. These deaths are usually associated with inadequate protection and control of the airway, failure to detect disruption of the breathing mechanism, major internal haemorrhage in the head, chest or abdomen, or multiple lesser injuries. Almost all injuries of this type are **treatable** by currently available medical and surgical procedures. For these patients, the interval between injury and initiation of effective treatment is critical to the probability of recovery, hence the concept of the 'golden hour'.

The third peak of late deaths consists of those patients who die days or weeks after injury, typically while in an ICU. The cause of death in 80% of this group is either systemic sepsis or multiple organ failure, often as a result of **inadequate or delayed initial resuscitation and management**.

INITIAL ASSESSMENT AND MANAGEMENT

In this book and on the CCrISP course, we are concerned primarily with the management of the injured patient after the golden hour, in the setting of the ward, ICU or HDU. However, to emphasise the concept of a continuum of care for the multiply injured patient, it is appropriate here to summarise the events that will have taken place before the patient is admitted from the emergency department.

The concept of initial assessment and early management in the pre-hospital and emergency department setting is dealt with elsewhere (MRCS Learning Course). The approach to the patient during the initial assessment period demands a system, and the one in most common use is that developed by the American College of Surgeons and taught by the Surgical Royal Colleges of England, Ireland and Australasia – the Advanced Trauma Life Support (ATLS®) system (see Table 15.1).

Table 15.1 *ATLS strategy*

Rapid primary survey
Concurrent resuscitation
Secondary survey
Definitive care

ATLS defines one effective strategy for the assessment and resuscitation of an injured person: initial assessment requires assessment and provision of resuscitation in five areas, denoted ABCDE (see Table 15.2). The purpose of the exercise is to identify what is killing the patient and in what order, and to **do something** about it.

Table 15.2 *Primary survey*

A	Airway and cervical spine control
B	Breathing and ventilation
C	Circulation and haemorrhage control
D	Disability: neurological status
E	Exposure and environmental control

Resuscitation is therefore conducted concurrently with assessment. Once the most urgent and life-threatening problems have been dealt with, a secondary survey can be performed in the form of a systematic examination, inspecting and investigating the patient from head to toe.

ADMISSION PATHWAYS

The fate of the patient with multiple injuries will often be decided by the efficiency of the early measures described above. Ideally, by the time the patient is admitted to the ward or an HDU or ICU, they should have been assessed accurately for injury extent and severity, resuscitation measures should have been effected, and a clear plan for future activities should have been decided. However, life is rarely this simple. A number of admission pathways for multiply injured patients may be defined. The following are likely scenarios:

- The patient is assessed fully and accurately, resuscitated adequately and investigated before admission to an appropriate ward prior to institution of definitive care measures. Unforeseen life-threatening problems in this scenario are unusual, but there is still a significant potential for less severe injuries to have been missed or overlooked early on.
- The patient is assessed fully and accurately and initially resuscitated but requires immediate surgical intervention to maintain successful resuscitation. In this scenario, full investigation will be deferred until completion of surgical resuscitation and may well reveal other previously undetected or overshadowed lesions that may require subsequent surgical interventions, planned or emergent. These patients are typically in danger and require ongoing, multidisciplinary critical care management.
- The patient is assessed inadequately, resuscitated poorly and not investigated fully. Such a process may not be recognised, and the patient may be admitted to a general ward and typically will deteriorate some time after arrival. This often occurs when managing elderly patients or those with compounding illness, when staff are busy or when the severity of injury has not been appreciated fully.
- The patient's poor condition is recognised but the cause is unknown. Under these circumstances, the patient may be admitted directly to an ICU bed for further management.

THE MULTIPLY INJURED PATIENT IN DANGER

The patient with multiple injuries may face continuing hazards in the hours following admission from the accident and emergency (A&E) department. The question often asked is under whose care should a patient with multiple injuries be admitted? A patient with an occult abdominal injury and obvious multiple fractures may not do well on an orthopaedic ward. The problem, then, is to define patients **at risk**.

One answer is to admit all patients with injury to multiple body systems to an HDU, where a multidisciplinary care plan can be effected. Ideally, even patients who have apparently been well stabilised should spend a period in such an environment. Patients are usually seen initially (in A&E) by adequate numbers of adequately trained staff. When patients are moved on, often to the radiology department, those not involved centrally tend to drift away. Particularly when initial investigations fail to show a convincing or expected diagnosis, immediate multidisciplinary reassessment (and further stabilisation) is needed, yet the necessary staff may have left. Safe practice after the golden hour therefore depends on all involved parties contributing positively and effectively from the outset and continuing to do so until a definitive plan is under way. **Do not 'leave it to others'!**

From your own perspective, working as a junior surgeon, patients described in the second and third scenarios above are at most danger, but such dangers may not be immediately obvious to you. Remember the scenarios are merely examples: there are many others that could be cited and, indeed, you may well have already encountered a similar situation.

> ### Practice point
> The main purpose of this instruction period is to raise your index of suspicion and improve your management skills when confronted with the multiply injured.

ASSESSMENT OF THE MULTIPLY INJURED FOLLOWING HOSPITAL ADMISSION

The hallmark of good trauma management is the recognition that trauma is a dynamic illness requiring **continuing re-evaluation**. In addition, you must not assume that assessments carried out before the patient's admission have been complete: be suspicious.

The following approach is recommended:

1 Repeat the primary survey phase to detect any evidence of deterioration during transfer to the ward or HDU.

> **PITFALL**
> If the patient is found to be unstable on admission to the ward/HDU, you must return to the beginning of the primary survey and work through it until you find the reason for the patient's continuing instability or deterioration. You must not proceed to a lengthy full and detailed systematic examination until the patient's condition is stabilised. If the patient fails to stabilise, you are missing something, or urgent surgical intervention may be indicated to deal with ongoing haemorrhage in a body cavity; this will be discussed in detail later.

2 Reassess the effect of any earlier interventions. Included here are reassessment of airway manoeuvres, the siting of chest drains or other endocatheters, and the response to intravenous fluids. Recheck the haemoglobin.

3 If the patient appears stable, then proceed to a complete secondary survey. Although this may have been performed before admission, it is unlikely to have been sufficiently comprehensive.

4 Important information about the mechanism of injury as well as the patient's past medical history frequently comes to light hours or even days after injury. This information may yield clues about **missed injuries** as well as complications that may occur. Some examples (by no means exhaustive) are:
   - Patient unrestrained and windscreen shattered in bull's-eye manner: consider missed injury to cervical spine, facial bones, myocardial contusion (if steering wheel damaged), pelvic and lower-limb injury.
   - More than 20 cm of inward front bumper deformation: this is statistically associated with increased likelihood of serious injury to the torso, pelvis, femoral shafts and knees.
   - Paramedics report that the vehicle went out of control for no apparent reason: consider associated illnesses, such as MI, cerebral ischaemic episode, epilepsy or diabetes mellitus.
   - Relatives disclose drug history: consider effects of, for example, anticoagulants, beta-blockers and insulin.

5 Systematic reassessment. You will now conduct a full and thorough top-to-toe assessment of the patient, consider further investigations and begin to formulate a definitive management plan, which may involve specialists from multiple disciplines. You will need to consider priorities at each stage as you proceed.

The method of conducting a secondary survey is covered in detail in the MRCS and ATLS courses. The purpose here is to restate the importance of repeated assessments, to emphasise pitfalls and to indicate where reassessment in the HDU setting differs from a secondary survey in the resuscitation room of an A&E department. Check and double-check: make your own full assessment, including looking at X-rays.

Even if the patient had a secondary survey previously, they should be re-examined fully as soon as possible on arrival in the HDU or ward (effectively a tertiary survey). Further examinations will be carried out every few hours, and more frequently if the patient is unstable or if there is reason to suspect a missed injury, *ie* significant mechanism of injury or if the conscious level is altered or varying.

Start by returning to the airway, taking particular care to identify impending obstruction due to oedema following injuries or burns to the neck or face. If an artificial or surgical airway has been placed, check repeatedly for position and adequacy of the lumen and plan a definitive tracheostomy. Examination of the head and neck is frequently more revealing after the patient has been resuscitated and is awake and cooperating. Previously unsuspected injuries may be found on the face, mouth and eyes, and visual acuity should be tested. Bruises that were not initially apparent may be evident and point to underlying injury. Consider ordering appropriate X-rays and scans if previously unrecognised injury is detected or suspected.

Patients with multiple injuries should have had the cervical spine immobilised with a semi-rigid collar, sandbags and forehead tape and will have had a cross-table lateral X-ray taken in the resuscitation room. You will have to decide whether full immobilisation should continue and whether further investigation of the neck is appropriate. In a fully conscious and alert patient who gives a clear history, it may be possible to remove the collar if the available films have been cleared by a radiologist. If there is any suspicion of injury, based on the mechanism of injury, the patient's clinical state or X-ray appearance, the neck must remain immobilised until the patient has been reviewed by an appropriate specialist. Further investigation may be required, including CT or MRI. The timing of these investigations will be for debate in the light of other injuries – the point to emphasise is that unstable patients must not be sent to a CT or MRI suite for lengthy investigations. It is appropriate for you to examine the neck with the collar off provided the neck is immobilised manually during the procedure and the collar, sandbags and tape replaced on completion.

This is a convenient time to perform a full neurological assessment. This should include calculation of the Glasgow coma scale (GCS), assessment of pupil sizes and reaction, and a general examination of the motor and sensory functions of the limbs.

PITFALL: HYPOXIA

Before leaving the head, face and neck, you must ensure that the patient is breathing high concentrations of oxygen and continue this until proven unnecessary.

You should now examine the chest. Examination of the chest is directed at identifying pneumo- or haemothorax, chest-wall injury and non-ventilating sections of the lung, injuries that may have been missed during initial assessment earlier. Following adequate chest films, it may now be appropriate to perform chest drainage for simple pneumothorax, for example. If tubes or needles are already in situ, their position and adequacy must be checked and further X-rays ordered or definitive treatment planned.

Adequacy of circulation is now confirmed. Take note of earlier measures, note the number, position and size of cannulae, check how much fluid has been given, and note whether blood or blood products were used. It is important to check how much blood, if any, is available in the blood bank. Take note of initial findings (pulse/blood pressure/pulse pressure) when the patient arrived in the resuscitation room, check the response to fluid challenges and note the patient's status on arrival on the HDU/ward. These data may well give you a clear view of how the patient is going to behave in the hours ahead. The presence initially of unexplained hypotension or a minimal or transient response to fluid resuscitation is a strong pointer to a missed injury. It is also appropriate at this stage to check the status of any wounds detected earlier.

Remember that your patient may be in transit to the operating theatre or pending further investigation before planned surgical intervention and much can go wrong during the waiting period. You do not need to remove dressings, but you should check for uncontrolled bleeding or recurrence of bleeding. If a urinary catheter is in situ, arrange to have hourly or half-hourly measurements of output. A continuing urinary output of more than 50 ml/h is usually a good indicator that fluid resuscitation is adequate.

> **Practice point**
> • Act on positive signs.
> • Re-evaluate negative signs.

You should carefully assess the abdomen and pelvis, a major reservoir for occult blood loss.

Examination of the abdomen is always more revealing when the patient is awake and co-operative, and will include full exposure, palpation for tenderness or peritonism, and auscultation. Examination is not complete until the flanks, back, lower chest and pelvis have been seen and palpated. Look for wounds, bruising and abrasions, which may overlie a hidden injury. Rectal and vaginal examinations should be performed but are easily overlooked. The absence of bowel sounds is common after blunt trauma and does not necessarily indicate significant intra-abdominal trauma, but it is reassuring when these return, and the presence or absence of normal bowel activity is important in the planning of nutritional support.

Signs are unreliable, especially when negative, but re-evaluation can be of help. Clear signs of peritonism, gastrointestinal tract damage (bleeding, increased amylase level) or hypotension in the presence of abdominal injury require senior surgical assessment. Although surgical management is becoming more conservative, this decision must still be made by the surgeon who would operate. Equivocal cases require investigation. Be particularly aware that secondary rupture of viscera (eg bowel or gall bladder) can present several days

down the line, when an organ that had its blood supply damaged at the primary injury becomes gangrenous and finally ruptures.

> **PITFALL**
> If you suspect the presence of a previously undetected intra-abdominal lesion, or if there is continuing unexplained hypotension, you must summon appropriate assistance.

Examination of the pelvis in a multiply injured or unconscious patient is vital. It should have been assessed and X-rayed while the patient was in A&E, but examination should be repeated. Unstable fractures of the pelvis are associated with massive ongoing haemorrhage. Operative fixation or angiographic embolisation is an emergency procedure and may take precedence over other interventions. Summon orthopaedic help early.

Injuries to the limbs (especially the feet) are often missed during initial resuscitation and may become apparent only hours or days later. Unfortunately, it is the non-management of these injuries that often causes functional disability in the long term and, therefore, it is imperative that every bone in the arms and legs is examined carefully, particularly in the unconscious or ventilated patient. Although it is important to assess the limbs in an unconscious patient, be aware that the evaluation cannot be regarded as complete until the patient is awake and co-operating. You should note such considerations in the patient's chart. Limb assessment can best be done in the sequence of look, feel, move. Act on suspicion and investigate radiologically. In the presence of fractures, the limbs must be assessed for signs of compartment syndrome, and dressings or casts released as required.

> **PITFALL**
> Do not miss a compartment syndrome: always consider the possibility in the presence of fractures, severe soft-tissue injury or crushing.

Finally, all tubes, drains, access lines, catheters and dressings should be checked and rechecked to ensure they are placed correctly and functioning normally and that there is no sign of infection supervening. Remember: this is a medical rather than a nursing responsibility.

CHART REVIEW

Regularly review all recorded data, ideally on a major trauma sheet, similar to those used on the ICU. Take particular note of vital signs, beginning with respiratory function – tachypnoea or hypoxia must be explained and prompts re-examination of the chest and further CXRs. Impending shock, evidenced by increasing tachycardia, oliguria and developing hypotension, will need rapid resuscitation and investigation for the cause, which might be occult bleeding into the abdomen, pelvis or chest, or from a previously undetected long-bone fracture(s), a cardiac injury or sepsis. A downward trend noticed on review of repeated GCS suggests an intracranial lesion and requires urgent CT.

PITFALL: HYPOTENSION IS A LATE SIGN

Many patients – not just the young and fit – can maintain blood pressure until a late stage, where they collapse suddenly. Think perfusion!

Available results and simple investigations

A full blood count is helpful, but remember that haemoglobin concentration is no guide to bleeding or adequacy of resuscitation in the acute phase. However, results from repeated investigations over time may be helpful, and results may be useful to gauge the requirement for red cell replacement hours after the initial resuscitation. White cell count is always raised after multiple injury, but an increasing neutrophil leucocytosis or a sudden fall in white cell count may indicate major sepsis. After significant volumes of fluid replacement, clotting may be abnormal, and after massive transfusion disseminated intravascular coagulation may develop. Urea, creatinine and electrolyte levels are primarily a guide to renal function, which may be

deranged following neglected hypovolaemia, massive transfusion or metabolite load associated with crush injury.

Arterial blood gases are essential if there is any question of adequacy of oxygenation or ventilation after a chest or abdominal injury, and to ensure the PCO_2 is not elevated in a patient with head injury. It may also be extremely useful if metabolic acidosis is present, as this is evidence of inadequate cellular perfusion, which requires explanation. If there has been an episode of profound shock, one may find that the acidosis gets worse initially with good resuscitation, as unperfused capillary beds are reperfused (washout phenomenon), but one needs to be cautious in attributing any worsening to this: the patient may simply be getting worse.

ECG monitoring is required if there is any evidence of cardiac injury, as defined by significant rhythm abnormalities or 'current of injury' abnormalities on a 12-lead ECG.

Once the patient is stable in the ward or HDU, all the X-rays performed should be carefully reviewed for skeletal injury, and all areas of tenderness or dysfunction identified during the examination should now be X-rayed.

Review of the drug chart

Patients with open injuries should be given necessary tetanus prophylaxis at the earliest possible opportunity. Patients with open fractures must be treated with a broad-spectrum antibiotic, usually a cephalosporin. Consider thrombosis prophylaxis, such as subcutaneous or low-molecular-weight heparin, since DVT is common following trauma.

Finally, ensure that the patient is charted properly for any regular drugs, including pre-injury regimens if applicable. Patients normally on steroid agents will always require steroid replacement following injury.

DAILY MANAGEMENT PLAN (STABLE PATIENTS ONLY)

If there are multiple teams involved in ongoing management, then someone has to take day-to-day responsibility for overall management. It will probably be you, or a career registrar like you. You will be the ringmaster.

Prescribe **oxygen** when it is required. If the patient is unable to maintain adequate oxygenation, consider assisted ventilation sooner rather than later (see Chapter 3). Prescribe appropriate fluids and blood product replacement, taking account of earlier deficits as well as normal daily requirements. Most fit, young patients are best managed well hydrated with above-normal urine output, but take care with the elderly, who may have a diminished circulatory reserve, and patients with head injuries. Maintenance of an accurate input/output chart is important.

Consider a **nutrition plan** from the first post-injury day. All patients with multiple injuries are catabolic and benefit from appropriate early feeding to support higher catabolic rate, tissue repair and immune function. The aim is to prevent rapid loss of muscle bulk and prolonged subsequent rehabilitation. Arrange **physiotherapy** early, particularly for the chest but also for limb, spinal or head injury, in consultation with orthopaedic surgeons or neurosurgeons. Consider what physiotherapy can be provided for early immobilisation of the limbs. Most patients are best managed sitting up in bed.

Finally, make plans with the various members of the multidisciplinary team concerning ongoing management of drains, splints, catheters, external fixators and traction devices.

Practice point

With multidisciplinary teams involved in management, there is a need to define who is in overall charge of the patient. As a supporting specialist, attend and review frequently and support the co-ordinating team by active involvement.

SPECIFIC INVESTIGATIONS

The patient who is unstable or deteriorating, whether initially or subsequently, must be treated as rapidly as possible in order to prevent death or halt developing complications. There may be time for investigation, but if there is hypotension then immediate transfer to the operating theatre because surgical resuscitation may be needed. Stable patients can be investigated more safely and in more detail.

CT head scanning and intracranial pressure monitoring

The patient with a head injury and a GCS of eight or less requires immediate control of airway and ventilation followed by a head scan, as does a patient with a falling GCS of 13 or less, or with lateralising signs (pupils or limbs). The purpose of this CT scan is to identify a surgically treatable lesion such as an extradural or subdural haematoma. Evacuation of an expanding haematoma should be done as a matter of urgency and may require inter-hospital transfer (see later). A patient in the above group who does not have a surgically correctable lesion is likely to have raised intracranial pressure (ICP) due to intracranial mass effect (haematoma, swelling, etc). As the mass enlarges, ICP rises and cerebral blood flow falls, putting the patient at risk of ischaemic brain injury, a secondary and **usually preventable** injury. Such an injury will be exacerbated by systemic hypoperfusion or hypoxia, and these must be corrected. Management under these circumstances is best conducted in the ICU, and you must arrange the patient's transfer immediately. In the patient with a severe head injury who has no surgically treatable lesion or who is post-surgery, ICP monitoring should be considered.

Cerebral perfusion pressure (CPP) is the difference between the mean arterial pressure (MAP) and the ICP. The formula is thus $CPP = MAP - ICP$. The two aims of modern ICU management of severe head injury with raised ICP are the preservation of adequate CPP and the reduction of ICP. The goal is a CPP of 70 mmHg or greater and an ICP of less than 25 mmHg. Control of ICP is at least as important as the maintenance of CPP, as the risk of poor outcome increases in a patient who has had significantly raised ICP, even if the CPP has been maintained.

In the setting of an ICU, ICP should be measured directly with an ICP monitor.

ICP can be reduced by:

- *Nursing the patient at a 30-degree head-up tilt:* this allows both arterial perfusion and adequate venous drainage of the brain.
- *Avoidance of neck compression:* this allows adequate venous drainage by avoidance of compression of the jugular veins. If a cervical spine fracture is suspected, the patient can be nursed with sandbags each side of the head to stabilize the neck, with the rigid collar left on but undone.

The collar can then be tightened during any movement of the patient, without the need to keep taking the collar on and off.

- *Sedation and paralysis:* sedation allows the patient to be ventilated appropriately and avoids the patient coughing and straining on the ventilator. This is vital to avoid surges in ICP. Paralysis reduces the level of sedation required to keep a patient stable on a ventilator but can produce problems of its own, such as a predisposition to infection.
- *Temperature:* pyrexia is associated with increased ICP and must be avoided if possible with the help of antipyretics (*eg* paracetamol). Conversely, trials of deliberate hypothermia have yielded conflicting results.
- *Ventilation* to ensure that PCO_2 is maintained at low normal values (around 4–4.5 kPa). Lower values of PCO_2 may lead to inadequate blood flow to the brain and are associated with a worse outcome. Hyperventilation to 3.5 kPa may be useful as a short-term emergency measure until alternative surgical or medical treatments can be instituted.
- *Mannitol and furosemide (frusemide):* hyperosmolar agents such as mannitol induce an 'osmotic' diuresis. This is thought to be the mechanism by which they reduce the ICP and cerebral water content. Mannitol is an effective but temporary method of reducing ICP. It can be used more than once, but it is less effective each time it is used; consequently, timing of administration must be discussed with the neurosurgical team (who should be involved by now). Furosemide also causes a rapid decrease in ICP; although it may work as a diuretic, a more important mechanism may be that furosemide crosses the blood–brain barrier, acts upon cell membranes to limit the uptake of chloride and sodium ions, and thus limits brain swelling.
- *Other agents:* trials of the use of barbiturates and corticosteroids in patients with severe head injury are continuing. You should use these agents only as part of your unit's protocol or when directed to do so by the neurosurgical team. A number of other agents are currently undergoing clinical trials.
- *External ventricular drainage:* this provides a means not only to measure ICP but also to treat secondary obstructive hydrocephalus and raised ICP itself to some extent.
- *Surgical decompression:* there is some evidence accumulating that decompression of the cranial cavity by removal of a bone flap until the period of maximum swelling has passed (three to five days) may benefit otherwise healthy young patients if performed early before ICP rises too high and brain damage is incurred.

Chest investigations

Bronchoscopy is frequently useful in the management of chest injuries as it can both diagnose easily missed lesions such as bronchial or tracheal injuries and treat mucus plugging. Echocardiography can be used to investigate cardiac injuries, particularly to exclude **pericardial tamponade**, although 'FAST' (focused abdominal sonography in trauma) ultrasound scanning in the emergency department is rapidly superseding this (see below). Echocardiography is also useful in experienced hands for investigating thoracic aortic injury. The benchmark investigation for aortic injury is still aortography, but the accuracy and shorter time required for helical CT may see this become the procedure of choice in the next few years. Clearly, intrathoracic injuries that are causing ongoing ventilatory or haemodynamic instability and not controlled by intubation and ventilation or tube drainage require surgical intervention to prevent shock or secondary injury to other organs. Involve the thoracic team members early.

Abdominal investigations

The abdomen of a severely injured patient frequently presents a difficult diagnostic problem. Intra-abdominal injury must be excluded in the patient with unexplained hypovolaemia. If there is instability, FAST scanning will answer the question as to whether there is a significant amount of blood (fluid) in the abdomen. The logical response to a positive FAST scan is to proceed to laparotomy.

However, if time permits and facilities allow, it may be better to answer a different set of questions: 'What is the organ injury?' and 'Can I continue non-operative management safely?' Rapid helical CT answers these questions best, but this algorithm applies only to the stable patient.

Helical CT also offers the advantage that it can be performed at the same time as scanning of other regions, such as the head. It does require the patient to go to the radiology department for a possibly lengthy period, during which the patient may suffer a circulatory collapse if the degree of injury and adequacy of resuscitation are misjudged.

> **PITFALL**
> - Multiple injury patients must not be sent for CT unless they are stabilised.
> - Unstable patients may die in the CT suite.
> - Even stable injured patients need planned safe transfer to and continued close monitoring in the CT scanner.

Diagnostic peritoneal lavage (DPL) is a very sensitive but less specific investigation. It answers a similar question to FAST and is therefore rapidly being superseded by the quicker and less invasive investigation. Its advantage is that it may be performed in the safety of the critical care environment with minimal equipment or if suitable ultrasound is unavailable. Its main disadvantages are its relative oversensitivity for minor hepatic injuries and that it makes subsequent CT scan interpretation difficult.

DPL/FAST should be reserved for the patient with unexplained hypovolaemia in whom urgency or the severity of shock precludes travel to the CT suite. It is important to appreciate that the technique of FAST is a disciplined one, and this is not a 'diagnostic ultrasound of the abdomen' such as would be performed in a radiology department. Such a test has been shown to be inferior to CT in defining injury after abdominal trauma.

Other investigations of the abdomen, including intravenous urography (IVU), cystography and urethrography, should be performed when there is suspicion of renal tract injuries. CT with oral contrast is used to exclude duodenal rupture.

CT scanning is occasionally necessary in order to define the nature of fractures, particularly complex fractures of the spine, pelvis and acetabulum. CT or MRI may be useful in the assessment of patients with suspected cervical spine injury who have normal or equivocal plain X-rays. CT or MRI is essential for the investigation of spinal injury to identify the likely degree of nerve damage and to assess the possible benefits of surgical decompression and stabilisation of spinal fractures.

SURGICAL TREATMENT OF THE PATIENT WITH MULTIPLE INJURIES

Management of a severely injured patient requires a high level of physiological support, but it usually also requires appropriately timed aggressive surgical intervention. This should be performed **as early as possible** to prevent secondary injury or to prevent long-term functional disability.

Surgery to treat major ongoing bleeding in the chest or abdomen should be performed on admission as part of resuscitation, but some patients will 'escape the net', arrive on the ward or HDU, and the decision will fall to you to arrange immediate transfer to the operating theatre. Do not delay in the false belief that patients with ongoing bleeding must be 'stabilised' before they can be operated on safely. Such patients cannot be stabilised without operation, and more and more fluid simply pushes them down the path to coagulopathy, acidosis and hypothermia, from which survival is increasingly unlikely.

In recent years, there has been a trend towards non-operative treatment of stable injuries of the liver and spleen, but this decision **must** be made at a senior level and close observation is needed. If complex and bleeding liver injuries are found at surgery, then packing and transfer to a specialist unit is appropriate. This established treatment is now being extended to the concept of damage-control surgery, where the shocked and perhaps coagulopathic victims of multiple trauma undergo limited early surgery restricted to making the patient safe and better able to survive definitive treatment 24–48 hours later.

At the other end of the spectrum, occasional patients need immediate surgery. Thoracotomy in A&E is indicated only for patients with penetrating thoracic injury who arrest in hospital or who will clearly not survive to reach theatre. It is pointless in exsanguinating blunt chest trauma, but occasionally aortic clamping or internal massage will salvage the patient exsanguinating from thoracic or abdominal haemorrhage. It is much better to get the patient to theatre before this state is reached.

Decompression of intracerebral haematoma is performed as soon as the diagnosis is confirmed and the patient has been fully perfused and oxygenated. This usually follows a period in a critical care environment.

The management of skeletal injuries should be planned from the beginning, and early stabilisation of fractures considered. Open fractures always require immediate surgery (within eight hours) for debridement and internal or external fixation. Closed long-bone and major joint fractures should be fixed early by external fixation, intramedullary nailing, or open reduction and internal fixation with plates and screws. This controls bleeding and pain, and hence shock, allows early physiotherapy and makes nursing easier. Early fixation also appears to reduce the risk of later sepsis and organ failure. In the unstable patient with multiple long-bone fractures, external fixators can be applied very quickly for the same reasons. In practice, most patients require urgent rather than emergency surgery and will be admitted to the HDU or ICU pending preoperative preparation and investigation. It may be appropriate in some instances to deliberately avoid intervention or to delay for several days to avoid the 'second hit'.

ABDOMINAL COMPARTMENT SYNDROME

Patients who have suffered a severe episode of shock, particularly those who have been coagulopathic, hypothermic and acidotic and have undergone a damage-control procedure, are at risk of progressive swelling and oedema of the abdominal contents and rising IAP.

Measurement of IAP is best achieved by measuring bladder pressure via the urinary catheter. The drainage tube is clamped and 50–100 ml of sterile saline instilled. Pressure tubing is connected to a transducer or manometer zeroed at the pubic symphysis and connected to the catheter either by needle puncture of an injection port or T-junction connector.

Impaired mucosal blood flow has been shown with elevations of IAP to as little as $13–15\,cmH_2O$, and progressive problems ensue with subsequent increases. Most authorities would consider a level of $25\,cmH_2O$ as a point where abdominal compartment syndrome is likely if the pressure is unrelieved. The consequences are renal failure, gut ischaemia, high airway pressures and impaired ventilation and, if recognised, should prompt a decompression by reopening the abdomen and placing a mesh or some other temporary closure until the swelling subsides. The most important message is not to attempt to close an abdomen that is already tight. This condition can also occur in severe burns, even when the abdomen has not been opened.

INTER-HOSPITAL TRANSFER

In most large institutions, inter-hospital transfer is uncommon. However, there are occasions when a patient's needs exceed the capacity of a particular institution to meet them. The patient's need for transfer must be recognised early, ideally in the resuscitation room. The protocols for transferring and receiving patients are covered in detail in the ATLS manual. Suffice it to emphasise that patients who remain unstable despite resuscitation **will not survive transfer**, and this may mandate the movement of a specialist team to the patient. Patients being transferred must be accompanied by appropriately skilled attendants and may require intensive life support en route. The receiving hospital must be notified and agree to transfer, and all documents and investigations relating to the patient must be sent. Intra-hospital transfer can also be dangerous – this should also be a planned, monitored and accompanied event.

CONCLUSIONS

Management of the patient with multiple injuries presents a major challenge and involves many of the principles taught in other parts of this course. More than any other surgical disease, multiple injuries require the co-ordinated care of a multidisciplinary team and appropriate use of all levels of care from the ward, HDU through to the ICU. Surgery must be timed carefully, and teams from different specialties must co-ordinate their efforts to be effective. These patients are challenging, but most are young and fit: if managed well, most can be expected to make a good recovery.

SUMMARY

- Reassess from the beginning – ABCs onward.
- Re-evaluate clinically and monitor closely.
- Consult at an early stage.
- Support colleagues actively when they are in overall charge.
- Early definitive treatment improves outcome.

Appendix

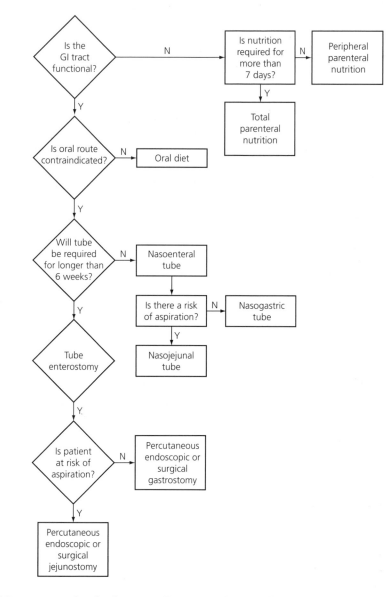

An algorithm for deciding on appropriate feeding route. (Reproduced from Hill, G.L., Disorders of Nutrition and Metabolism in Clinical Surgery, 1992, by permission of the publisher Churchill Livingstone.)

Index

Bold page numbers refer to figures and *italic* page numbers indicate tables.